Earl Mindell, R.Ph., Ph.D. is also the author of

Earl Mindell's Anti-Aging Bible
Earl Mindell's Soy Miracle Cookbook
Earl Mindell's Soy Miracle
Earl Mindell's Food as Medicine
Earl Mindell's Herb Bible

EARL MINDELL'S SECRET REMEDIES

The Essential Guide to Treating Common Ailments with Vitamins, Minerals, Herbs, and Other Cutting-Edge Supplements

Earl Mindell, R.Ph., Ph.D.

A Fireside Book
PUBLISHED BY SIMON & SCHUSTER

FIRESIDE
Rockefeller Center
1230 Avenue of the Americas
New York, NY 10020

Designed by Jenny Dossin

Manufactured in the United States of America

1   3   5   7   9   10   8   6   4   2

Library of Congress Cataloging-in-Publication Data
Mindell, Earl.
[Secret remedies]
Earl Mindell's secret remedies : the essential guide
to treating common ailments with vitamins, minerals, herbs,
and other cutting-edge supplements / Earl Mindell.
p.   cm.
"A Fireside book."
Includes bibliographical references and index.
1. Diet therapy—Popular works. 2. Dietary supplements—Popular works.
I. Title.
RM217.M563   1997
615.8'54—dc21   96-49168
                                           CIP

ISBN 0-684-81827-2

This book is dedicated to my wife, Gail, our children, Alanna and Evan, our parents and friends, and the many wonderful people who have helped me throughout the years, and to the health of all peoples worldwide.

Acknowledgments

I wish to express my deep and lasting appreciation to my friends and associates who have assisted me with this book. I would like to thank Angela Osborne for her dedication and hard work throughout this entire project. I would also like to thank Harald Segal, Ph.D.; Bernard Bubman, R.Ph.; Edward Powell, R.Ph.; Sal Messineo, Pharm.D.; Allan Kashin, R.Ph.; Arnold Fox, M.D.; Donald Cruden, O.D.; Nathan Sperling, D.D.S.; Ray Faltinsky; and Kevin Fournier. A special thanks to Carol Colman Gerber and my editor, Caroline Sutton, for their help. Also, much thanks to my agent Richard Curtis for all his support throughout the years.

Contents

Secret Remedies

Since the publication in 1979 of my first book, *Earl Mindell's Vitamin Bible*, I have traveled widely throughout the United States speaking about health issues in general and about supplements in particular. I am always surprised at the number of people who patiently wait in line to ask me questions after my talks. Often the questions are ones that I have heard before. Here is just a sample of the ones that I am frequently asked:

- Are there any natural remedies for migraine headaches?
- Are there any supplements that can help me to lose weight?
- What should I be taking for an enlarged prostate gland?
- Is there anything I can do to prevent breast cancer?
- I have terrible PMS. Are there any supplements that can help?
- Is there anything that you can recommend for chronic fatigue syndrome?
- What can I take to calm my nerves?
- Are there any vitamins that can bolster my immune system?
- Are there any supplements that can relieve hot flashes?

In *Earl Mindell's Secret Remedies,* you will find answers to these questions and many more. Here you will find specific, easy-to-follow instructions about how to prevent and treat more than fifty common health problems through the use of supplements that are sold over the counter at natural-food stores, pharmacies, and your neighborhood supermarket.

Early in my career as a pharmacist and master herbalist, I became frustrated that the healthcare system paid vastly more attention to the treatment of disease than its prevention. In the United States, I was one of the earliest advocates of the use of supplements, and I am proud that my books, including *The Herb Bible* and the *Antiaging Bible*, have helped introduce millions of readers to the role supplements can play in maintaining robust health and in treating disease.

As a pharmacist, I understand that conventional drug therapy occupies a very important role in health care. There is no disputing that antibiotics have saved countless lives, that chemotherapy has revolutionized the treatment of cancer, and that drugs that lower blood pressure have prevented countless heart attacks. But these drugs must be used judiciously. For example, antibiotics should only be prescribed sparingly. If they are overused—as they often are—they can be rendered ineffective or, even worse, can give rise to antibiotic-resistant bacteria. For the most common ailments—cold and flu—which are caused by viral infections, antibiotics are virtually useless. The overuse of antibiotics has become a growing and serious problem. As this book goes to press, the Centers for Disease Control (CDC) in Atlanta is embarking on a public service campaign to discourage the indiscriminate use of antibiotics. The CDC notes that since 1980, the use of antibiotics has soared by 40 percent, and there has been a simultaneous 25 percent rise in the growth of antibiotic-resistant bacteria and fungi. If this trend continues, antibiotics may pose a greater threat to our health than the infections they are designed to defeat.

Moreover, many of the drugs that are commonly prescribed for ailments such as high blood pressure, depression, and sleep disorders cause very unpleasant side effects that can seriously interfere with the quality of life. The good news is that in many cases, for many ailments, the correct supplements can do the job as well if not better than conventional drug therapy with few if any side effects. There are also times when supplements can enhance the effect of conventional drugs, thereby hastening recovery. Finally, and perhaps most important, supplements can be a useful tool in helping to prevent the onset of many diseases in the first place.

Secret Remedies will make it easier than ever to stay healthy, vital, and strong. Based on cutting-edge medical research being performed at leading medical institutions in the U.S. and abroad including the National Cancer Institute and the National Institute on Aging, *Secret Remedies* alerts readers to the latest and most important breakthroughs in the field of supplements. In recent years, there has been an explosion in information on how vitamins, minerals, herbs, hormones, amino acids, and other supplements can help prevent disease as well as maintain overall health and vigor. Recent findings include:

- **Vitamin E is heart healthy.** A study of more than eleven thousand men and women ages sixty-seven to one hundred five performed by the National Institute on Aging showed that those who took Vitamin E supplements were half as likely to die from heart disease as those taking no supplements at all.

- **Calcium lowers blood pressure.** According to a major study on children's health (the Framingham Children Study) those who consumed the most calcium had the lowest blood pressures. In adults, calcium has been shown to lower the risk of developing high blood pressure.

- **Folic acid protects against cancer.** Folic acid, a B vitamin that can prevent serious birth defects in developing fetuses, is now believed to help prevent cervical cancer.

- **Ginkgo improves brain function.** This ancient herb can help improve circulation throughout the body including the brain and, studies show, can enhance mental function.

- **Gluthatione boosts immunity.** This amino acid is produced within the cells of the body. A recent study shows that a glutathione supplement can bolster immunity in older adults, thereby improving their resistance to infection.

This is just a small sample of the work being done on vitamins, minerals, herbs, and other supplements that I report on in this book.

There are many different kinds of supplements; some may be familiar to you, some may not. Here is a brief description of the supplements that I discuss in *Secret Remedies*, as well as a definition of some common terms.

Antioxidants—Many of the supplements I write about are *antioxidants*, substances that protect the body from damage by free radicals. The antioxidant theory of disease was proposed by scientist Denham Harman several decades ago. Dr. Harman believed that aging was actually a form of "rusting," that like old cars left out in the rain, our bodies can form rust that prevents them from operating efficiently. The "rust" is actually caused by exposure to oxygen. We all know that oxygen is essential for life and, without oxygen, our bodies would cease functioning. Oxygen is instrumental in *metabolism*, the ability of cells to make energy. Yet, in the wrong form, oxygen can be very dangerous. In the process of making energy, cells produce substances called *free radicals*, which are highly unstable oxygen atoms. Because they are so unstable, free radicals are likely to bind with other atoms and, when they do, they give off energy. In the body, free radicals transfer their energy to the cells of body tissues, which can cause great damage. The human body produces many different types of antioxidants that help to tame these free radicals before they can do their damage; these include vitamin E, glutathione, and coenzyme Q10, among others. As we age, however, we produce fewer antioxidants, thus allowing free radicals to run amuck. It is believed that, over time, free radicals slowly and insidiously damage important tissues and organs, including our arteries, our hearts, the cartilage between bones, and even our brains. Damage by free radicals is believed to be a major cause of many different diseases, including heart disease, Alzheimer's disease, cancer, Parkinson's disease, and arthritis. By replenishing our supply of antioxidants, we may be able to inhibit the activity of free radicals, thereby forestalling the aging process and the diseases that are associated with aging.

Phytochemicals—A general term referring to thousands of compounds naturally occurring in plant foods including vitamins, minerals, and *phytoestrogens* (hormonelike substances), which have been shown to have a protective effect against certain common diseases, including cancer, heart disease, diabetes, high blood pressure, osteoporosis, and infection. Some better known phytochemicals include:

* **Carotenoids.** More than six hundred compounds found in green leafy vegetables, or orange fruits and vegetables, foods such as broccoli, cantaloupe, pumpkin, mangoes, and peaches. The best known carotenoid is betacarotene, but there are others of equal importance including alphacarotene and lycopene (found in tomatoes).

* **Bioflavonoids.** More than five hundred compounds that give fruits and vegetables their color. At one time, bioflavonoids were considered to be little more than food dye, but today many of these compounds are being investigated for their anticancer and disease-fighting properties. Bioflavonoids have been used by natural healers for years to treat asthma and allergy; some asthma medications are based on synthetic versions of these compounds. Recent studies have found that some bioflavonoids are antiviral and can strengthen capillaries (tiny blood vessels), which if weakened, can promote bruising and internal hemorrhaging.

* **Phytoestrogens.** Hormonelike compounds found in plants that are similar to the estrogen produced by the the body, but with some very important differences. Like real estrogen, plant estrogens bind to estro-

gen receptors in cells, thereby preventing real estrogen from binding to these cells. Unlike real estrogen, however, plant estrogens do not stimulate cell growth, therefore, plant estrogens are believed to inhibit the growth of tumors that would normally be stimulated to grow by real estrogen.

Vitamins—Vitamins are organic substances that are essential for life. They are found in food derived from both animals and plants. Although ancient physicians did not know that vitamins existed, they sensed that food contained substances that had therapeutic value. For example, more than two thousand years ago, folk healers prescribed calves' liver to treat night blindness. What these healers did not know is that liver is an excellent source of vitamin A, which is essential for good vision. The word *vitamin* was first used in 1912 by a Polish scientist, Casimir Funk, who discovered that the hull of a polished rice grain contained an organic substance that could prevent beri beri. (*Vita* is Latin for life; *amine* means an organic-hydrogen compound.) Although he did not know it at the time, Funk had discovered vitamin B. Since then, many more vitamins have been discovered, and we now more fully understand the important role they play in our bodies.

Vitamins are called *micronutrients* because the amounts that are required for normal functioning are minuscule, yet vitamins perform very important tasks. Among other things, vitamins help us digest our food, fight infection, and manufacture new cells. With rare exceptions, vitamins cannot be manufactured by the body, and must be obtained from food or supplements. Severe vitamin deficiencies will result in serious illnesses, such as *rickets* (lack of B vitamins) or *scurvy* (lack of vitamin C.) Even a modest deficiency in certain vitamins, however, can have a profound effect on health. Vitamins help our bodies operate at peak efficiency and, if we are short of key vitamins, over time, we will feel the negative effects.

There are two kinds of vitamins: water soluble and fat soluble. *Water-soluble vitamins* are not stored in the body and excess amounts are washed out in urine. On the other hand, fat-soluble vitamins (A,D,E, and K) are stored in the liver. Fat-soluble vitamins cannot be properly absorbed by the body unless we consume an adequate supply of fat and minerals.

Water-soluble vitamins are usually measured in milligrams or micrograms. Fat-soluble vitamins are usually measured in International Units or IUs.

Minerals—Minerals are naturally occurring chemical elements found throughout the human body in the bones, muscles, teeth, blood and nerve cells. Minerals help to maintain a normal water balance within the body, and are involved in virtually every activity from immune function to the beating of our hearts. Deficiencies in minerals such as calcium, potassium, and magnesium can result in high blood pressure, thinning of the bone (osteoporosis), and irregular heart beat. Essential minerals (calcium, magnesium, potassium, and sodium) are required in amounts ranging from several hundred milligrams to more than 1 gram (1000 mg.). Trace minerals (such as selenium, iron, and chromium) are required in much smaller quantities, and are often measured in micrograms or millions of a gram.

Herbs—Herbs are plants that are used for food, flavoring, and/or for medicinal purposes. In fact, herbs have been used to prevent or treat disease for thousands of years. Moreover, nearly 50 percent of the thousands of commercial drugs commonly used and prescribed today are derived from a plant source or contain chemical imitations of a plant compound. For example, digitalis, which is used to treat heart arrhythmias, is derived from the foxglove plant. Quinone, a famous treatment for malaria, is made from the bark of the cinchona tree. Even penicillin, the "founding father" of the antibiotic revolution, is actually derived from a mold, an organism produced by a fungus.

Until recently, most herbs were only available in plant form and were difficult to use. Today, most of the important healing herbs are available in capsules, teas, and extracts at natural-food stores.

Amino acids—Amino acids are organic compounds that are the building blocks of all proteins. There are twenty-two different amino acids; 14 of these can be made by the body but eight others, called *essential amino acids,* must be obtained through food or supplements. Some important amino acids within the body do not form proteins, they are referred to as nonprotein amino acids (such as taurine and L-carnitine.)

Hormones—Hormones are chemical messengers within the body that tell cells what to do. Hormones control a wide range of bodily functions including reproduction, sex drive, sleep, immunity, and digestion, to the ability to think and talk. The decline in certain key hormones, notably DHEA and melatonin, are believed to be instrumental in the aging process and are now being explored as treatments for specific diseases.

Probiotic—*Probiotic* is a general term used for supplements that do not kill bacteria directly (like antibiotics), but rather bolster the body's own defenses against disease. Probiotics include various vitamins and herbs that stimulate immune function, including echinacea and acidophilus. Although antibiotics can be very effective in wiping out an infection, in the process they can kill off "good" bacteria within the intestine that help aid in digestion, and can cause stomach upset and vaginal yeast infections. Besides, antibiotics are not invincible. In fact, they can be rendered defenseless against antibiotic resistant bacteria.

Enzyme—An *enzyme* is a protein found in living cells that brings about chemical changes. A *coenzyme* works with an enzyme to produce a particular reaction. Some of the supplements that I discuss are either enzymes or coenzymes.

How to Take Supplements

Unless otherwise noted, you should take your supplements after meals, since a full stomach enables your body to better absorb the nutrients. Some supplements, however, such as digestive enzymes, should be taken prior to meals, and in these rare instances, I will note the exception. Common sense dictates that supplements that induce sleep (such as melatonin) or have a tranquilizing effect (such as valerian) should only be taken in the appropriate circumstances. It is of course advisable not to drive or operate machinery after taking any supplement that makes you drowsy.

Supplements come in a wide variety of brands and forms, ranging from capsules to pills to sublingual pills (which are dissolved under the tongue) to teas to creams and gels. In some cases, I specify a particular form for a particular supplement. For example, I prefer the sublingual form of vitamin B12 because it is the one that is best absorbed by the body. I also recommend calcium ascorbate for vitamin C because it is the form that I have found to be gentlest on the stomach, and the dry form of vitamin E because I feel that it is the most potent. I want to stress, however, that there is nothing wrong with the other forms of these supplements, simply that these are the forms that I myself prefer.

Supplements should be stored in a cool, dry place out of direct sunlight. Some supplements should be refrigerated: Be sure to read the label for precise instructions.

As good as supplements are, they are no substitute for a healthy lifestyle and good nutrition. It is still essential to eat a good diet, to exercise regularly, and to get enough sleep. If you smoke or abuse drugs or alcohol, supplements cannot negate the effects of these dangerous practices.

Although most supplements are safe, some can nevertheless be toxic at high levels. **You can avoid most potential problems by sticking to the recommended dose.**

Not all supplements are for all people. For example, if you are pregnant, you should be very cautious about taking any medication, including supplements, unless it is prescribed by your physician. Here are some other caveats.

Combination Multisupplements

I am frequently asked whether it is better to take each supplement individually, or to take a combination multisupplement containing several vitamins, minerals, and herbs all in one pill or capsule. Indeed, there are many excellent combination multisupplement formulas on the market that are geared for specific problems. For example, there are multisupplements with potent antioxidants; multisupplements specifically geared for prostate health and multisupplements for women suffering from PMS or looking to relieve menopausal symptoms. As long as the multisupplement you choose contains the appropriate vitamins, minerals and herbs, there is no reason not to use it. Certainly, taking one pill is a lot easier (and sometimes more economical) than taking a dozen different ones. Therefore, whenever possible, I recommend combination multisupplements for those who want to use them. When it is not possible, however, I still recommend taking individual supplements, or augmenting a combination multisupplement with other supplements.

Caution: If you have a preexisting condition and are being treated by a physician or natural healer, do not selfmedicate. Check with your physician or healer before adding any supplements to your regimen. If you have allergies, check with your physician before using any herbs. Depending on what you are allergic to, some may be helpful, but some may actually aggravate your condition.

Vitamin A: Pregnant women should not take more than 5,000 IU of vitamin A daily; very high doses of vitamin A have been linked to birth defects.

B6: This vitamin should not be taken by anyone under L-dopa treatment for Parkinson's disease.

Vitamin C. If you have diabetes, discuss the proper dosage of vitamin C with your doctor. Too high a dose could interfere with your medication.

Vitamin E: If you are taking aspirin or other blood thinners or have a vitamin K deficiency, check with your doctor before taking vitamin E, which is also a blood thinner. If you have an overactive thyroid, diabetes, high blood pressure, or rheumatic heart disease, build up your dose of vitamin E slowly. Start with a very low dose of 50-100 IU, and gradually increase your dose by 100 IU each month until you reach between 400–800 IU.

Ephedra: This herb, a natural antihistamine, has long been used as a treatment for colds, flu, and respiratory problems. In fact, it contains two compounds, ephedrine and pseudoephedrine, that are used in many over-the-counter cold and allergy medications. If used judiciously, ephedra is safe for most people. If you take too much ephedra, however, it can produce rapid heart beat, and speedlike symptoms that can be very dangerous, even fatal. Unfortunately, there have been reports of ephedra abuse by some teenagers who are looking to get high. If you use ephedra, you should do so only for a very limited time under the supervision of your physician and/or natural healer. (People with diabetes or high blood pressure should avoid ephedra, as should pregnant women.)

Ginseng: Ginseng can raise blood pressure in some people. If you have high blood pressure, check with your physician or natural healer before using ginseng.

Magnesium and potassium: Magnesium and potassium supplements should not be taken by people with kidney disease.

Niacin (Vitamin B3): This vitamin (which is often prescribed for high blood cholesterol) should be used with caution by anyone with severe diabetes, glaucoma, peptic ulcers, impaired liver function, or gout. If you have any of these conditions, check with your doctor before taking niacin. If you do use niacin, niacinamide is the preferred form; it reduces side effects such as the hot flush that can often result from niacin supplements.

St. John's wort: This natural antidepressant can cause sensitivity to sunlight. If you are taking St. John's wort, avoid exposure to the sun.

Acne

Countless teenagers have been made miserable by acne, but so have countless adults. Although acne typically strikes between the ages of eighteen and twenty-four, it can occur at any age, and often does.

Acne is a disorder of the sebaceous glands in the skin. The sebaceous glands secrete a substance called *sebum*, a fatty lubricant that is secreted through pores and hair follicles, which are most abundant on the face and scalp. Acne occurs when the pores become clogged with sebum. When sebum is exposed to oxygen, it turns black and forms *blackheads*, external plugs consisting of sebum and dead cells which may be attacked by bacteria, causing pus-filled inflammations, or pimples. (In contrast, whiteheads are pus-filled skin inflammations that are not necessarily acne related.)

In teenagers, acne is typically caused by a hormonal imbalance, and the same is true for adults. Sufferers of adult acne often have higher than normal levels of male hormones, which can stimulate the production of sebum.

Salicylic acid, sulfur, and resorcinol are nonprescription lotions, creams, and gels that are used to treat mild acne. Although they can't prevent new pimples, they can cause existing ones to dry and peel.

Stronger antibiotic solutions or lotions and oral antibiotics are available by prescription and can inhibit bacterial growth and decrease the number of inflamed pimples. In many cases, natural remedies should help reduce the signs of acne but if they don't, your doctor can tell you about other options.

There are several supplements that can help to keep acne under control.

Vitamins

Vitamin A—Some of the hottest new treatments for acne are actually derived from Vitamin A, which should not be surprising. Vitamin A has long been touted as the vitamin for beautiful skin. In fact, a number of medical studies demonstrate that high doses of vitamin A can correct

21

cystic (boil-like) acne, but since high doses may be toxic, consultation with a dermatologist is essential. *Retinoic acid,* a synthetic form of vitamin A, is also an effective topical treatment of cystic-type acne but, again, you need to get a prescription for this treatment from your physician. (High doses of vitamin A can cause birth defects, so it should *never* be used by pregnant women.)

Vitamin C—As early as 1954, a researcher gave large doses of vitamin C to fifty-three acne patients; forty-three improved on an 8-ounce glass of citrus juice served twice daily and 3,000 mg of vitamin C. Today, we know that vitamin C is essential for the formation of *collagen,* the stuff that binds together the cells of connective tissue; it is also essential for the maintenance of healthy skin.

Minerals

Zinc and selenium—Pimples can easily become infected, which can cause both pain and scarring. Zinc and selenium are two immune-enhancing minerals that can help fight against infection.

Helpful Herbs

Evening primrose oil—This substance is high in GLA (gamma-linoleic acid) a natural antiinflammatory, and may be helpful in treating teenage acne. Evening primrose oil is available in capsules.

Grapeseed—Sold under several different brand names, grapeseed contains *bioflavonoids,* substances that are related to vitamin C and have been reported to be highly effective acne fighters. Why do these compounds work? Skin cell nourishment depends on healthy blood circulating in the dermis layer. Collagen, one of the primary components of the dermis, determines the skin's strength, elasticity, and smoothness. Collagen cannot be made without vitamin C, and grapeseed and other bioflavonoids enhance vitamin C in its healing power. Grapeseed extract is available in capsules or tablets.

Acidophilus—Known as the "good bacteria," for its ability to control yeast infections, it has also been found to be an effective addition to the acne-fighting arsenal. Acidophilus is found in yogurt and is available in liquid and capsules. (If you eat yogurt, beware of sugar-filled yogurt that does not contain live acidophilus cultures and may be counterproductive.)

Vitex—Some women may develop acne each month prior to their menstrual periods, when hormone levels are fluctuating. Vitex, also called *chaste tree fruit*, imitates the action of some hormones, such as estrogen and progesterone, and has been used for thousands of years to remedy a number of hormonal irregularities. It has been successfully used to treat acne and premenstrual herpes on the lip. For external use.

Garlic—One of nature's most versatile bulbs. It not only enhances the flavor of many foods, but its chock-full of vitamin A, B and C, calcium, potassium, iron, carotene, germanium, and selenium, plus countless biologically active compound agents. Most of all, it contains the amino acid *allicin* (short for allyl disulfide) which, when used externally as an oil, helps reverse acne.

Jewelweed—This extract is a Native American treatment for poison ivy and other topical irritants. Creams made from this herb can reduce redness, irritation, and inflammation, but will not necessarily prevent irritation.

Bee pollen—Contains a rich concentration of nucleic acids. When applied topically, these substances penetrate the skin surface where they nourish epidermal cells and tissues and have a cleansing effect on acne. Bee pollen can also be taken orally.

Calendula—An essential oil that can be used for many purposes and is included in many skin care preparations. It is an excellent cleanser.

Tea tree oil—Apply a drop of tea tree oil to the lesions twice a day. Applying alternating hot and cold compresses to the skin can help to open pores and eliminate excess oil.

Personal Advice

Although it is widely believed that fatty foods can trigger acne, this is not the case. In fact, you may be surprised to learn that salt and the iodine in salt may be the more troubling culprit. Avoid salty foods:

Watch your intake of chips, fries, and processed foods. Keep the skin scrupulously clean, but take it easy with harsh skin cleansers. Squeezing pimples can trigger inflammation, turning a relatively benign blackhead or whitehead into a pustule, which can leave a scar. This treatment is commonly applied during professional facials; it might be wise to ask your cosmetologist to skip this procedure.

Stress affects every part of our body, so it makes sense that it can affect our skin. Meditation, exercise aroma therapy, and the use of herbal oils to massage and clean the skin can all help lessen tension and help restore that glow to the skin that is often lost during those stressful teen years.

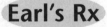

Earl's Rx

If you have acne, try these supplements for beautiful skin.

Acidophilus: One tablespoon of acidophilus liquid or one to three capsules one-half hour before eating, up to three times daily.

Betacarotene: Take 25,000 IU daily.

Bee pollen: Bee-pollen cream can be applied directly to the lesions up to three times daily.

Selenium: One or two capsules or tablets (100–200 mcg.) daily.

Zinc: One 15–50 mg. capsule or tablet daily.

Vitamin C: Two 500 mg. capsules or tablets of calcium ascorbate daily. This the gentlest form of vitamin C for your stomach.

Grapeseed extract: Up to three 100 mg. capsules or tablets daily.

Evening primrose oil: One to three 500 mg. capsules daily.

Vitex (for women): One to three capsules daily.

Alcohol Abuse

Too much alcohol can cause severe vitamin and mineral deficiencies. Drinking in excess can increase the risk of developing heart disease, high blood pressure, chronic liver disease, some forms of cancer, neurological diseases, nutritional deficiencies, and many other disorders.

In our society, alcohol is such a commonly used substance that we often forget that it is actually a drug, and a potent one at that. Alcohol works by depressing the central nervous system. Since ancient times, alcohol has been used for medicinal purposes, as part of religious ceremonies, and for recreation.

Like many other drugs, alcohol is absorbed through the stomach, and is then metabolized by the liver, processed by the kidneys, and secreted in the urine. Small amounts are also processed through the lungs and exhaled in the breath. The effects of alcohol on the human body depend on the amount of alcohol consumed, the rate at which it is consumed, and whether or not it is being drunk on an empty stomach (in which case its inebriating effects are felt almost instantly).

For most people, a drink or two will make them feel relaxed and enhance their sense of wellbeing by repressing their inhibitions. Heavy alcohol use is typically defined as more than two drinks daily. (One drink equals 4 ounces of wine, 8 ounces of beer, or 1 shot of hard liquor.) As far as I'm concerned, however, the less alcohol consumed the better, because it can sap the body of vital nutrients. For example, alcohol impairs calcium and vitamin C absorption, two nutrients that, among other things, are essential for strong bones, which is why women who consume more than two glasses of alcohol daily are at high risk of developing osteoporosis. An occasional glass of wine is fine, but I certainly do not recommend drinking on a regular basis, and if you do drink, I would stop at one drink.

For the alcoholic, however, alcohol is sheer poison and even one drink is one too many. The alcoholic is not a "social drinker," but someone who has a need to drink that is overpowering and destructive. Alcoholics Anonymous aptly defines alcoholism as "an obsession of the mind coupled with an allergy of the body."

Treating alcoholism is a complex undertaking and addiction specialists are best qualified to handle the care and management of the true alcoholic. Of course, getting the alcoholic to stop drinking would be the first priority in treating the disease. New research into a very old herb may produce a treatment that can actually lessen the desire to drink.

The Kudzu Story

Two active ingredients from the root of the kudzu vine, *Pueraria lobata*, have been identified and tested in animals at Harvard Medical School. Researchers Ming-Wing Keung and Bert Vallee injected Syrian golden hamsters with an extract of the root of one of two of its previously isolated active ingredients, daidzin and daidzein. They then gave the hamsters a choice between plain water and alcohol mixed with water. The hamsters who had previously preferred the mixed drink opted for the plain water more than 50 percent of the time.

Researchers attribute the change in preference for plain water to the ability of the root to lessen the desire for alcohol. Scientists have yet to demonstrate that kudzu will have the same affect on humans, but they do know it has been used by traditional Chinese healers since 200 B.C. to treat alcohol abuse.

In China and Japan, healers brew the plant into a medicinal tea. Although up to a liter must be drunk every day to achieve the desired effect, the root extract has reportedly become available recently in tablet form in China. Chinese doctors report that after approximately two to four weeks of treatment, up to 80 percent of patients no longer have a craving for alcohol, with no adverse reactions.

Replacing the Lost Nutrients

When consumed in large amounts, alcohol ravages the body with toxins that destroy vitamins and minerals necessary for good health.

Glutathione—This combination of three amino acids—glutamate, glycine and cysteine—is a powerful antioxidant that helps protect the body from poisons.

Thiamine—Thiamine deficiency is very common among alcoholics because it can be destroyed by alcohol. Vitamin B1 (thiamine) is available in supplement form and is found in ham, pork, sunflower seeds, peanuts, fortified cereals, green peas, artichoke, corn, melon, and pompano fish.

Herbs

Milk thistle—One of the oldest known herbal medicines, it has been used for over two hundred years to treat various liver disorders. One use of milk thistle that has emerged from research is its ability to stimulate the regeneration of tissue and function in the livers of alcohol abusers by stimulating cellular protein synthesis.

Turmeric—This spice been revered in India for thousands of years, and researchers there have conducted most of the research into the healing chemical it contains: *curcumin*. One animal study showed that curcumin has a protective effect on liver tissue exposed to liver-damaging alcohol. Although the FDA generally regards the spice as safe, turmeric should be used in medicinal amounts only in consultation with a physician.

Personal Advice

One more reason not to drink to excess: Alcohol can be very fattening. In fact, someone who has a drink or two daily can be consuming hundreds of extra calories. Here's the double whammy—since alcohol slows down the metabolism, it makes it more difficult for the body to burn fat.

For the moderate drinker who suffers from the occasional hangover, forget the idea that coffee is the cure-all. In fact, after the initial burst of energy one gets from caffeine, coffee only increases fatigue and nausea.

Try an herbal tea, such as mint, before going to bed after a night of imbibing. The menthol in mint may relax the smooth muscle lining of the digestive tract, acting as an antispasmodic. Chamomile is another good remedy because of its mild, tranquilizing effect. A tea of equal parts kudzu root and fresh ginger root (both available at health-food stores) has an antispasmodic effect on the lining of the stomach and may lessen the affects of a night on the town.

If you can look at food the next day, try starchy carbohydrates like cereal, which will help keep your body fueled as the liver attempts to rid itself of excess alcohol. Drinking lots of water (eight to ten glasses) will help the liver wash out the alcohol.

Finally, if you are a problem drinker, seek help from a qualified physician or natural healer that specializes in treating addictions.

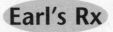

Earl's Rx

If you are trying to undo the harm inflicted by excessive drinking, I recommend the following regimen.

Milk thistle: One capsule up to three times daily.

Gluthathione: Up to three (500 mg.) gluthathione capsules on an empty stomach.

B complex: Two (50 mg.) capsules or tablets daily with food.

Vitamin C: Two (500 mg.) calcium ascorbate daily. Calcium absorbate is the form of vitamin C that is gentlest on the stomach.

Calcium: One (1000 mg.) capsule or tablet with 400 IU Vitamin D daily. In addition, when you take calcium, be sure to take 500 mg. of magnesium for every 1000 mg. of calcium consumed to maintain the body's normal mineral balance.

Allergies

35 million people in the United States suffer from various allergies.

Just when the snowstorms of winter are fading from memory, and flu season ends, nature slams us with a one-two punch. Spring not only ushers in warm weather and sunshine, it also ushers in the hay-fever and allergy season.

The word *allergy* is of Greek origin and means "abnormal response." This response occurs when the body reacts abnormally to normally harmless substances such as pollen, dust, certain foods, drugs, animal fur, feathers, cosmetics, dyes, smoke, plants, molds, chemical pollution, insect stings, and even roach and animal excrement. (See "Asthma" for advice on how to dust- and mite-proof your environment.)

A chain reaction occurs when the immune system mistakes a benign substance for a dangerous foreign invader. The immune system goes into overdrive and produces an abundance of histamine; the histamine widens the hair-thin capillaries in the membrane, which increases blood flow; the increased blood flow results in swelling and congestion.

Allergens (the offending substances) also cause the white blood cells to produce the allergic antibody IgE. IgE molecules then travel through the bloodstream until they combine with mast cells (which line many blood vessels), or basophils (a type of white blood cell), which are the main storage sites for histamine and serotonin. The IgE allergic antibody then causes the capillaries to become "leaky," so that a watery fluid present in the blood escapes and causes a runny nose, sneezing, watery eyes, and nasal congestion.

Once allergens are identified, it makes sense to avoid foods and substances that cause the symptoms.

If allergens cannot be avoided, as with household dust and pollen, desensitization is sometimes beneficial. *Desensitization* involves injecting small amounts of the allergen under the skin over an extended period of time. After many such injections, the body may learn not to react to the substance.

Treatment of allergy symptoms generally consists of three types of medication: antihistamines, which block release of the histamines that cause swelling and congestion; anti-inflammatory agents such as cortisone; and decongestants such as ephedrine and phenylpropanolamine hydrochloride. However, it may be possible to wave good-bye to all those pharmaceuticals with a change in lifestyle and dietary habits, and with supplements that can help keep allergic reactions under control.

Vitamins

Quercetin—This member of the bioflavonoid family helps to stabilize the cell membranes of mast cells and basophils, thus preventing them from spilling their supply of histamine/serotonin into the surrounding blood and tissue. Yellow and red onions, shallots, Italian (summer) squash, broccoli, and blue-green algae are good sources of quercetin; it is also available as a food supplement. Quercetin is particularly effective when teamed with *bromelain,* an enzyme found in raw pineapple that is a potent anti-inflammatory.

Vitamin C—The same stress that triggers the release of histamine also increases the need for vitamin C, the body's natural defense against excessive histamine. Thus, allergies that cause the release of histamine also increase the need for vitamin C. In a recent study at Arizona State University, Carol Johnston, Ph.D., gave nine people vitamin C supplements for six weeks, beginning with 500 mg. daily and gradually increasing to 2,000 mg. per day. By the time the daily intake of vitamin C had peaked, histamine levels had dropped an average of 40 percent.

B-complex—The B-vitamin complex may also ease hay-fever symptoms. In particular, the B-vitamin pantothenic acid, with vitamin C, helps the body produce its own natural anti-inflammatory, cortisone.

Herbs

Echinacea—Known commonly as *purple coneflower,* it promotes health by boosting and balancing the immune system.

Ginkgo biloba—May help prevent bronchial constriction typical in asthma that often accompanies severe allergies. Since asthma is often triggered by allergies, ginkgo may be a valuable allergy-fighting herb.

Eyebright—Especially good for relieving the symptoms of hay fever, especially itchy eyes.

Nettle—A well-known folk remedy for hayfever and other allergies. It helps relieve inflammation and clear congestion.

Other Supplements

Omega-3 fatty acids—Omega-3 fatty-acid fish oils contain natural anti-inflammatory compounds. Omega-3 is found in fatty fish such as mackerel, albacore tuna, and salmon, as well as in flaxseed oil and purslane (a green leafy vegetable that can be used in salads.)

Personal Advice

Watch the stress—Stress places a heavy burden on the immune system, and allergic reactions are more likely to be triggered if the body is over-worked or overstressed. Exercise, meditation, yoga, and other stress-reducing techniques can ease the burden of stress on the immune system.

Earl's Rx

When allergies flare, try these supplements.

Vitamin C and pantothenic acid (part of B-complex): Equal amounts (1000 mg.) of vitamin C in the form of calcium ascorbate and pantothenic acid with food twice daily. The antihistamine action of vitamin C works especially well with the anti-inflammatory action of pantothenic acid. Many people report wonderful results with this combination.

Echinacea: Two or three (500 mg.) capsules daily for two weeks, then discontinue for two weeks. Resume for another two weeks, discontinue for two weeks, and continue the same pattern throughout allergy season. If you take echinacea constantly without a break, your body will build up a resistance against it and the herb will be rendered ineffective.

Quercetin and bromelain: Two 500 mg. combined capsules of quercetin and bromelain.

Ginkgo: Up to three 60 mg. capsules or tablets daily.

Alzheimer's Disease

Between 4 and 6 million Americans have Alzheimer's disease.

As the population ages, the number is expected to reach *14 million* by the year 2020.

Of all the diseases associated with aging, I believe that Alzheimer's disease is the one that is most feared, and for good reason. Alzheimer's disease is an irreversible deterioration of the areas of the brain that control reasoning and memory. As the disease progresses, the lives of Alzheimer's victims and their families are virtually turned upside down. Nerve-cell death causes a decline in ability to perform routine tasks, loss of cognition, impaired judgment, disorientation, personality change, and loss of language skills.

At the moment, there is no conclusive diagnostic test for Alzheimer's disease. In fact, diagnosis is only confirmed after death by studying the brain, which is marked by the accumulation of a protein called *beta amyloid*.

Scientists have come up with several intriguing theories as to the cause of this devastating disease. It is estimated that perhaps 15 percent of Alzheimer's may be due to an inherited gene, but not everyone who inherits a bad gene gets Alzheimer's, and the gene has not been found in many people who do have the disease.

Some researchers theorize that Alzheimer's may be caused by an overabundance of neurotoxins (nerve poisons), which specifically target nerve cells for death. Researchers also suspect that *glutamate*, a chemical in the brain, may kill nerve cells by increasing the calcium level within the cells or by strangling off the glucose supply to the cell, thus literally starving it to death.

Many researchers believe that *beta amyloid*, a protein buried in plaques that litter the brains of Alzheimer's victims, is a key player in the disease. This protein is also produced in virtually every cell in the body, which suggests that amyloid is not highly toxic itself, but may trigger Alzheimer's when it builds to a critical threshold in the brain. Scientists hope this discovery will enable them to rapidly screen potential drugs to see if they decrease amyloid output; however they still do not know if blocking amyloid will halt Alzheimer's.

One of the most controversial issues is the role that aluminum may or may not play in Alzheimer's. Some researchers have found high levels of aluminum in the brains of Alzheimer's patients, but others have not. To add to the confusion, Alzheimer's does not appear to be more common in communities with high levels of aluminum in their drinking water, nor do the millions of people who take aluminum-containing antacids seem to have higher rates of the disease. In my opinion, since we do not fully understand the role of aluminum, it makes sense to avoid unneccessary exposure. Aluminum is used in many products, including processed foods, antacids, toothpaste, foil, and antiperspirants. Read labels carefully, and try to buy products that are aluminum-free. Aluminum is also found in tea, but the aluminum in tea quickly passes through the body and usually is no problem. However, if you use lemon in your tea, the citric acid in the lemon can convert the aluminum into a salt that is readily absorbed by the body. The solution to this problem is easy: If you drink tea, do not use lemon.

Some researchers believe that inflammation is a key component of the disease. A study of elderly identical twins who were given either a nonsteroidal anti-inflammatory drug or a placebo showed that the twin taking the drug was less likely to get Alzheimer's than the twin who wasn't. The role that inflammation may play in Alzheimer's is not fully understood, but it is being investigated as a potential cause.

Given the fact that Alzheimer's is still such a mystery, it is difficult to devise a strategy to prevent this disease. However, there are some things that may be helpful.

Control Stress

Some studies suggest that the amount of stress experienced over a lifetime can add to the risk of getting Alzheimer's. Stress hormones, called *cortisol* or *glucocorticoids,* are pumped into the body and brain routinely in stressful situations. But in some older people the mental switch controlling stress seems to be stuck in the "on" position so that stress hormone levels are high all the time. These hormones impair the performance of cells in the *hippocampus,* the center of memory and cognition.

Does Estrogen Help?

Some studies show that women taking estrogen after menopause seem to have about half the risk of developing Alzheimer's. Researchers looked at information on estrogen-replacement therapy and other medical information for 8,879 women living in Leisure World retirement communities in southern California. Of the 2,418 women who died from 1981 to 1992, those who had used estrogen replacement therapy were 40 percent less likely to have had Alzheimer's than those who had not used estrogen. The fact that estrogen may reduce the risk of developing Alzheimer's disease is not surprising; there are estrogen receptors in the brain, especially in key memory centers, and several other studies have shown that estrogen replacement therapy can enhance both learning and memory.

If you do use estrogen, I recommend that you find a doctor who prescribes natural hormones, that is, hormones that are identical to the hormones produced by your body. Although these hormones are not aggressively marketed as synthetic hormones, they appear to be safer, and women who use them have fewer negative side effects. Estrogen, however, is not for everyone, and there are some women for whom it is not advisable.

There are also supplements that can help you to stay smart and sharp.

Antioxidants

As I have noted earlier, antioxidants protect cells against damage inflicted by free radicals, those overactive oxygen molecules formed in the body from the oxygen we breath that can destroy healthy cells. Brain tissue is particularly vulnerable to attack by free radicals. There is compelling evidence that free-radical activity may be increased in Alzheimer's patients and, if this is the case, it is likely that antioxidants will have a protective effect. Two studies have reported that people with Alzheimer's have low levels of vitamin E, one of the most potent of all antioxidants. Clinical investigations on older adults using nutritional supplements of various mixtures of vitamins E, C, coenzyme Q10, B6, and selenium, have provided some encouraging results in delaying the progression of Alzheimer's. If you are not already taking some combination of antioxidants daily, you should!

Minerals

Zinc—According to a 1990 study reported in *Family Practice News*, zinc deficiency may be related to Alzheimer's. The mineral has been found to be in low levels in the hippocampus (memory center) of the brain in Alzheimer's patients. In addition, zinc seems to prevent deposits of lead and other toxic metals, the formation of which can lead to tangles in the brain characteristic of Alzheimer's.

Magnesium—A deficiency of this mineral is also thought to be a factor in Alzheimer's disease. Magnesium helps to protect against stress and age-related brain-cell deterioration.

Amino Acids

L-carnitine—Short for *acetyl-l-carnitine*, L-carnitine is an amino acid produced by every cell in the body and, according to European studies, appears to slow down the mental deterioration that accompanies Alzheimer's. Curiously, a just-completed large clinical trial in the U.S. did not confirm that L-carnitine is effective against Alzheimer's— researchers are at a loss to explain how a study could be so positive in one country (Italy) and not in another. Since L-carnitine also provides excellent protection against heart disease, however, I feel it makes good sense to take it as a hedge against Alzheimer's and other diseases of aging.

Helpful Hormones

Melatonin—This "miracle" hormone produced in the pineal gland ensures that the levels of other vital hormones stay within a normal range in response to environmental change. For instance, when we are exposed to prolonged stress, our adrenal glands produce stress hormones called *corticosteroids*. Exposure over time to high levels of corticosteroids can cause damage to many of our organs and has been linked to Alzheimer's.

Melatonin may also help Alzheimer's patients to recover their normal sleep patterns—a boon to caregivers and patients alike.

Pregnenolone—This hormone, which is now being sold over-the-counter, has been shown to be a potent memory enhancer. Pregnenolone is produced both in the brain and in the adrenal cortex, the glands that sit above the kidneys. Like other hormones such as melatonin, pregnenolone production declines with age. By the time we are seventy-five, we are making 60 percent less pregnenolone than we did in our thirties, and many researchers believe that the loss of pregnenolone and other hormones may be why our brains begin to age. Pregnenolone is hardly the new kid on the block. In fact, as far back as the mid-1940s, a group of industrial psychologists tested pregnenolone on students and workers and discovered that it markedly improved their ability to learn and remember difficult tasks. Today, it is being used by enlightened doctors and alternative healers to help prevent memory loss in older people and to keep Alzheimer's symptoms at bay.

Herbs

Ginkgo biloba—Ginkgo biloba exerts a positive effect on the vascular system. Recent studies of ginkgo biloba extract show that it increases blood flow to the brain and lower extremities. It has been shown to improve memory and to relieve signs of senility, including Alzheimer's, probably due to the increased blood flow to the brain. Again, preliminary studies show that ginkgo biloba is most effective in delaying mental deterioration in the early stage of the disease, but does not reverse it.

Personal Advice

Use it or lose it—Studies in China, Finland, France, Israel, Italy, Sweden, and the United States show that the more educated you are, the less likely you are to get Alzheimer's. The possible explanation? The brain is just like the rest of the body, and if you "exercise" your brain, you stimulate the cells to work harder and become stronger. Thus, those with more education who continue to have an active interest in learning are less likely to contract Alzheimer's.

B is for brain power—A shortage of B vitamins, notably B12, can cause Alzheimer-type symptoms. B12 deficiency is quite common among the elderly, and anyone showing signs of senile dementia should take 1000 mg. of B12 sublingually (dissolved under the tongue) daily. In some cases, B12 injections may be necessary. I have seen people perk up considerably with this treatment, and the confusion and memory loss quickly disappears.

Earl's Rx

Here are some super supplements for your brain.

Antioxidants: There are numerous antioxidant formulas on the market. Be sure to find one that includes the basics for your brain: vitamins E, C, and selenium and ginkgo biloba.

L-carnitine: One 500–1000 mg. tablet daily on an empty stomach.

Magnesium: One 350–500 mg. tablet daily.

Pregnenolone: One or two 50 mg. capsules daily.

Melatonin: Take 1 mg. sublingual tablet (dissolve under the tongue) at bedtime. (If you wake up groggy, you may need to reduce your dose by breaking the tablet in half.)

Zinc: One 15–50 mg. capsule or tablet daily.

Coenzyme Q10: 30–100 mg. daily.

Anemia

Iron-deficiency anemia is the most common nutritional disease in the world.

Women are particularly vulnerable to iron-deficiency anemia.

Do you tire easily? Do you have difficulty concentrating? Are you always cold? These are all symptoms of *anemia,* a problem that results when the cells of the body are not getting enough oxygen. Anemia can be due to either a lack of hemoglobin, the substance that carries oxygen in the blood, or a shortage of red-blood cells, the special cells in which the hemoglobin is packaged and carried throughout the bloodstream.

The most common type of anemia is *iron-deficiency anemia.* Iron is essential for the production of hemoglobin, and if you are not getting enough of this mineral, you could have too few red-blood cells. Iron deficiency can result from chronic blood loss, lack of iron in the diet, impaired absorption of iron from the intestine, or an increased need for iron by the body, as in the case of pregnancy.

If you are feeling tired, run-down, and lack energy, don't self-diagnose and don't assume that gulping iron pills will make the problem go away. A definitive diagnosis can only be made by thorough testing by your physician or natural healer. If you are diagnosed with iron-deficiency anemia, your doctor will probably suggest that you increase the amount of iron-rich foods in your diet and/or take a daily supplement. The best food sources for *heme* iron, (the most absorbable form of iron) are lean meat and poultry, oysters, clams, and egg yolks. Nonheme iron, which is not as easily absorbed, is found in dark-green leafy vegetables; dark-red vegetables, such as red chard, beets, and red cabbage; dried fruit, beans, and whole grains and dried fruits. Sea vegetables like dulse and hiziki are also high in iron. Too much iron, however, has been implicated as a risk factor for heart disease. That is why I recommend that you have your blood-iron levels checked by your doctor to see if you are deficient before you begin adding iron-rich foods to your diet or taking iron supplements.

Anemia could also be the result of a defiency in key B vitamins, notably folic acid and vitamin B12, which are essential for the production of red-blood cells which carry the hemoglobin. A diet deficient in either of these vitamins could result in too few red-blood cells. Clearly, the right combination of diet and supplements can help to prevent anemia.

Vitamins

B12—Several studies have shown that many people over fifty are deficient in this vitamin. A deficiency in B12 will cause classic symptoms of anemia, such as excessive fatigue, mental confusion, and difficulty concentrating. For example, *pernicious anemia* is a chronic disease of older people in which the stomach fails to produce an enzyme needed for the absorption of vitamin B12, which is essential for the production of mature red-blood cells. B12 is primarily found in animal products, including meat and dairy foods, therefore vegetarians of any age who do not eat either meat or dairy products may be at risk of this form of anemia. Vegetarians who abstain from all animal products should take a B12 supplement. (If you don't eat meat, but still eat eggs and dairy foods, such as yogurt and cheese, you are probably getting enough B12.)

Vitamin C—Although iron from vegetables, fruit, and grains is more difficult for the body to absorb, vitamin C can improve absorption of these foods by as much as 85 percent. Taking a vitamin C supplement can enhance the effect of the iron that you are already getting from everyday foods.

Folic acid—This B vitamin, which has been shown to prevent birth defects if taken during pregnancy, is also essential for the production of red-blood cells, which will help prevent anemia. Folic acid is found in leafy green vegetables and whole grains, and is also available in tablets and capsules.

Minerals

Iron—Now that so many of us are cutting back on foods like red meat and liver to reduce our fat intake, we are inadvertently also cutting our intake of iron. For many people, especially women with heavy menstrual periods, an iron supplement to prevent anemia is necessary.

Herbs

Dong quai (Angelica sinensis)—rich in vitamins and minerals including B12, it may help prevent anemia.

Chive—These vegetables are rich in vitamin C and iron—a perfect combination, since vitamin C facilitates the absorption of iron. Chives should be eaten fresh.

Quinoa—A grain native to Bolivia and Peru, it is now being grown in the Rocky Mountains of Colorado. It is rich in all eight essential amino acids that form a complete protein, normally found only in red meat, eggs, and dairy products. Quinoa is much lower in calories and fat.

Rose hips, watercress, yellow dock root, burdock root, parsley, and **horsetail** are all iron boosters.

Personal Advice

If you feel fatigued, run-down, and lack energy, don't assume you are anemic. Get a physician's diagnosis, as iron-deficiency anemia can mask many different illnesses, some serious, some not. Women of child-bearing age should stay away from diets that drastically cut caloric intake without providing adequate nutrients.

Parents beware—Many teenage girls are particularly vulnerable to anemia because they are often dieting and, therefore, rarely get adequate vitamins and minerals. Dieting can be dangerous for several reasons, including the fact that it promotes nutritional deficiencies that can interfere with a girl's physical and mental functioning. Numerous studies have shown that iron-deficiency anemia can adversely affect a girl's ability to perform well at school. Obviously, if a girl is too tired to concentrate, she cannot do her best. Parents, however, are often too quick to dismiss the symptoms of anemia as typical teenage behavior, but that can be a mistake. I recommend that you err on the side of caution: If you suspect that your daughter is anemic, don't wait; take her to the doctor and get her help. It will make all the difference in how well she thinks and feels.

Earl's Rx

I think that these recommendations will help anyone with anemia. In particular, women who suffer from chronically cold hands and feet due to anemia have told me that they have "warmed up" with these supplements.

Iron: One 50–100 mg. tablet of heme iron daily with food.

Vitamin C: Two 500 mg. calcium ascorbate daily with food.

Folic acid: One 400 mcg. tablet daily.

Copper: One 2mg. tablet daily.

Vitamin B12: Take 800–1000 mcg. in sublingual form (dissolved under the tongue). The sublingual form of this vitamin is the one best absorbed by the body.

Anxiety and Stress

According to the American Academy of Family Physicians, more than *two-thirds* of all visits to doctors are due to stress-related ailments.

I recently had dinner with a friend of mine who is a doctor and asked her what was the most common complaint that she heard from her patients. "That's easy," she quickly replied, "anxiety."

What is so interesting about my friend's response is that she is not a psychiatrist, specializing in disorders of the mind, but an internist, specializing in the health of the various organ systems of the body. Her experience merely underscores the fact that the mind and the body are truly inseparable, and that what happens above the neck has a profound effect on what happens below it. If current studies are to be believed (such as the one I cite at the beginning of this section), anxiety is the number-one health problem facing Americans today.

Anxiety can stem from emotional, genetic, and even hormonal problems, but in most cases, it is caused by stress. Since these two problems are so closely linked, and since the treatments for both are virtually identical, I will discuss them together.

The term *stress* has become commonplace, but in reality, it was first used in connection with anxiety by Dr. Hans Selye in the 1930s. Dr. Selye was a brilliant *endocrinologist* (hormone specialist) who noticed that when animals were continually placed in frightening or unpleasant situations they experienced real and measurable physical changes in their bodies. For example, when rats were constantly placed in cold water or subjected to loud, annoying noises, they developed peptic ulcers. Up until Dr. Selye's study, the word stress was solely used by structural engineers to define the forces that can assault buildings, bridges, and other structures, such as earthquakes, high winds, and weight.

Stress is a wonderful word to describe what happens when we humans are assaulted by a difficult, frightening, unpleasant, or anxiety-provoking situation. The stress response, which is as old as humankind, is regulated by the *autonomic* or involuntary nervous system that controls such vital functions as the beating of our hearts. When we are faced with a scary, challenging, or nerve-wracking situation, the autonomic system goes on "automatic pilot," and triggers the cascade of events popularly known as the *flight-or-fight* response. It quite literally prepares us to flee a dangerous situation or fight for our lives. Our adrenal glands (located at the top of the kidneys) begin to pump out corticosteroids, or stress hormones, that rev our bodies up for action. Our blood pressure rises, our hearts pump faster, and the blood flow is diverted away from the abdomen to our legs, to prepare us to run faster. Our pupils dilate to let in more light so that we can see in the dark. We are geared up and ready for action. Now, if we were cave dwellers who frequently had to escape a dangerous predator or hunt for our every meal, we would use up our stress hormones in a burst of activity, and our bodies would quickly return to normal. For most of us, however, stress is quite a different experience. We are "assaulted" by demanding or rude bosses or clients, difficult family members, bills that need to be paid, and other stressors typical of modern life. Yet, since our bodies do not differentiate between one type of stress or another, when we experience stress of any kind, we go into overdrive. Unlike the prehistoric peoples who rapidly burned up the stress hormones that were being furiously pumped out by the adrenal glands, we do not, and these hormones linger in our bodies, which can cause substantial damage to vital organs and other bodily systems. In animals, studies have documented that constant exposure to stress hormones can, among other things, kill perfectly healthy heart cells, dampen the ability of the immune system to function normally, raise blood-sugar levels, and may even cause the thinning of bone, which can lead to osteoporosis. What is even more frightening is that several studies have shown that stress hormones can damage cells in the memory center of the brain in animals. In fact, human studies have shown that people who are under extreme stress perform less well on memory tests than those who are not. Clearly, stress not only makes us feel bad, but can have a profoundly devastating effect on our bodies.

It is not surprising that anxiety-relieving drugs such as Prozac have become so popular these days, or that medical journals are packed with advertisements touting the benefits of one tranquilizer over another. These drugs may be quick fixes, but they all can have unpleasant side effects, ranging from constipation to impotence to dry mouth—nor are the long-term effects of these mood altering drugs fully known. This is why more and more people are turning to natural remedies to help control stress and anxiety.

Vitamins

B-complex—B vitamins are nature's antidote to anxiety and stress. People who are low in B vitamins often show signs of depression, confusion, memory loss, and other symptoms of extreme anxiety. B vitamins work best together, which is why I recommend B-complex (B1, B2, B6, B12, and folic acid).

Minerals

Calcium and magnesium—When we are under stress, our blood-pressure levels rise, sometimes to dangerous levels. These two minerals can reduce blood pressure naturally, which will help our bodies withstand the potentially harmful effects of stress.

Herbs

St. John's wort—This herb, which is widely used in Europe as an antidepressant, is also good for reducing stress. Recently, according to a recent article published in the *British Medical Journal* researchers concluded that St. John's wort was as effective an antidepressant as many stronger prescription medications.

Siberian ginseng—For thousands of years, Asian healers have used ginseng as a tonic herb; that is, they do not necessarily prescribe it for particular ailments, rather they use it to maintain health and vigor. There are many different types of ginseng, and I personally prefer Siberian ginseng because, unlike some of the more potent forms, it does not cause insomnia. Ginseng also appears to help the body better withstand stresses of all kinds. For example, Russian researchers have found ginseng to be a stabilizer: That is, if blood pressure rises too high, ginseng lowers it, or if blood-sugar levels drop too low, ginseng spikes them back up to normal levels. Ginseng has also been shown to increase athletic endurance and performance, which is another sign that it kicks in when we are under stress.

Kava kava—This herb has been used in the treatment of nervous anxiety, insomnia, and restlessness. It is a natural tranquilizer, and can promote a feeling of well being.

Ginkgo biloba—This herb improves the circulation to the brain and can be an effective mood elevator in depression.

Chamomile—I end the day with a cup of chamomile tea. It has a pleasant, calming effect and is particularly good for a nervous stomach.

Natural Hormones

DHEA—This hormone, which is produced in the adrenal glands, brain, and skin, can help to control the damaging effects of stress hormones. As we age, our levels of DHEA decline, and by age forty we are producing half the amount of DHEA we did at age twenty. Not so coincidentally, as we age it takes longer for our bodies to recover from stress, and our levels of stress hormones remain higher for a longer period of time. Many animals studies have shown that DHEA supplements can prevent the normal physical damage caused by excess exposure to stress hormones, and there is strong evidence that it will do the same in humans. I feel that by age fifty, it makes good sense to restore DHEA to more youthful levels. For example, in a six-month study recently conducted at the University of San Diego, for the first three months thirteen men and seventeen women aged forty to seventy took a DHEA supplement sufficient to restore their blood levels back to those of young adults. For the next three months, the participants received a placebo. Neither the researchers nor the subjects knew who was taking DHEA or the placebo at any given time. The researchers found that when the participants were taking DHEA, they not only felt better, but said that they were better able to handle stress.

Melatonin—Melatonin is a hormone produced by the pineal, a tiny gland within the brain. Melatonin controls our sleep–wake cycle and is also a potent stress buster. Similar to DHEA, animal studies have shown that melatonin can regulate the negative effects of stress hormones by restoring them to more normal levels. An added bonus: Melatonin may help relieve insomnia caused by mild anxiety. By age sixty, we produce half the melatonin we did at age twenty, and many researchers believe that we need to restore melatonin back to youthful levels to maintain maximum health and longevity.

Personal Advice

Avoid caffeine—If you are under stress, caffeine will make you even more jittery. Switch to herbal, decaffeinated teas and decaffeinated coffee. Watch the cola drinks—they can be a hidden source of caffeine.

Exercise—As I explained, one of the reasons stress exacts such as steep toll from us is that stress hormones rev us up for action, but we do not follow it through by doing anything physical. Regular exercise is a great way to relieve stress and is a natural mood elevator.

Earl's Rx

B complex: One 50 mg. tablet twice daily with food.

St. John's Wort: One capsule up to three times daily.

Siberian ginseng: One capsule daily between meals.

Ginkgo biloba: One 60 mg. capsule or tablet up to three times daily.

Kava kava: One capsule up to three times daily.

DHEA: Take 25 mg. daily if you are over forty. Men over fifty can take 50 mg. daily. Women should not take more than 50 mg. unless it is done under a doctor's supervision.

Melatonin: Take 1 mg. sublingually (dissolved under the tongue) at bedtime.

Calcium and magnesium combination: One 500 mg. calcium and one 250 mg. magnesium tablet twice daily before meals. If you have difficulty sleeping, however, you can take calcium (1000 mg.) and magnesium (500 mg.) one-half hour before bedtime.

Arthritis

About 50 million people in the United States suffer from some form of arthritis. For more than 20 million of these people, the symptoms are severe enough to cause them to seek medical attention.

There is no known cure, but diet, medication, topical creams, and exercise can provide some relief.

Long before modern pharmacies with their shelves packed with literally row upon row of different brands of painkillers even existed, natural healers were devising strategies to treat one of the most common of all known diseases, arthritis. In fact, many of the remedies that are promoted by pharmaceutical companies today as state of the art are in fact either derived from or based on, time-proven remedies that have been used for centuries.

At least one in five Americans will experience the pain and discomfort of arthritis. There is no proven cure for this disease, but there are many different types of treatments that can help relieve symptoms. Before I discuss these treatments, let me first tell you a bit about the disease.

Arthritis is actually a general term for approximately one hundred diseases that produces either inflammation of connective tissue or degeneration of articular cartilage. *Cartilage* is the substance that lines the joints; it prevents the bone endings from rubbing together and allows the joints to move in a fluid way. As the cartilage gets worn down, the bones become exposed, resulting in pain, stiffness, and swelling in the joints. Although most forms of arthritis are related to aging, in reality, this disease can also strike the very young.

The two forms of arthritis that are most common are *osteoarthritis* and *rheumatoid arthritis*. Although they both result in the destruction of the joints, they are actually quite different diseases.

Osteoarthritis is also known as *degenerative arthritis* or, more popularly, as *wear-and-tear arthritis*. Osteoarthritis can affect all or some of the joints; symptoms include morning stiffness; which usually disappears within a half hour or so after rising, and pain and swelling of the joints (especially the fingers.)

In rheumatoid arthritis, the inner lining of the capsule that encases the joint, the *synovium,* becomes inflamed. The synovium grows and thereby destroys cartilage, bone, and adjacent structures. The widespread inflammatory process also involves other tissue, such as blood vessels, skin, nerves, and muscles. The result is painful joints, loss of mobility, and generalized soreness and depression.

Although we know the harm that arthritis can inflict on the body, we do not fully understand the cause of this disease. Damage inflicted by free radicals (unstable oxygen molecules) is believed to be responsible for many of the diseases of aging, including arthritis. Free radicals, in excess, can destroy *cell membranes,* the protective covering of cells. Humans have developed mechanisms that can protect against the formation of dangerous free radicals. Our bodies naturally produce many compounds that function as antioxidants and prevent oxidative damage to cells. They include vitamin E, glutathione, selenium, and vitamin C. Many experts now believe that by taking antioxidant supplements, we may be able to prevent the kind of free-radical damage that can lead to arthritic changes.

As I mentioned earlier, there is no magic bullet for arthritis. There are some effective treatments, but they are not without some risk. Noninfectious inflammatory arthritic diseases are typically treated with nonsteroidal anti-inflammatory drugs (NSAIDS) such as ibuprofen (Advil and Motrin) and naproxen (Naprosyn), that suppress inflammation by inhibiting synthesis of prostaglandins, hormonelike substances that cause inflammation. However, these drugs can be irritating to the stomach and can cause gastric bleeding. In addition, over time, their effectiveness can weaken. Other medications, such as cortisone, which are often prescribed for arthritis do relieve pain, but have such serious long-term side effects that they cannot be used indiscriminately. (Among other things, corticosteroids weaken the immune system, and can cause osteoporosis, the thinning of bone.) Therefore, I recommend that people first try to treat arthritis with time-proven natural cures that are safe, usually highly effective, and easy to use.

Herbs for External Use

Capsaicin—*Capsaicin* is the active ingredient of cayenne pepper, the fruit of *capsicum annum,* a shrubby tropical plant. Capsaicin is most helpful when applied topically as a cream to the aching joints of arthritis sufferers.

Eucalyptus oil—The oil of the eucalyptus plant provides relief from the pain of arthritis when rubbed on the skin. It increases blood flow to the area, thus producing a feeling of warmth.

Boswella serata—A cream derived from the *boswella serata* plant, long used by Indian healers, it is winning raves as an effective way to soothe aching joints.

Herbs for Internal Use

Bromelain—*Bromelain*, which is derived from the pineapple plant, is a well-known natural anti-inflammatory. Bromelain has been shown in clinical studies to reduce the need for corticosteroids, which are frequently prescribed for both osteoarthritis and rheumatic arthritis. Although corticosteroids are highly effective for relieving pain and inflammation they are not without side effects, including some potentially serious ones, such as high blood pressure, elevated cholesterol, and osteoporosis. Any natural and safe remedy such as bromelain that may reduce the need for corticosteroids should be tried. *also Dr. What*

Gamma linolenic acid—Found in evening primrose oil and borage seed oil, *gamma linolenic acid* is an omega-6 fatty acid similar to the omega-3 fatty acids found in fatty fish. Natural healers have long prescribed evening primrose oil to treat rheumatoid arthritis.

Asparagus, butcher's broom, tumeric, wild yams, yucca, Devil's claw, curry, angelica, barberry, black cohosh, juniper, licorice, and propolis (found in honey)—All contain steroidal-type compounds that may reduce inflammation caused by arthritis. Many of these herbs are included in preparations used to treat arthritis.

Siberian ginseng—Ginseng has been the subject of thousands of scientific studies and is known as the world's best antistress tonic. Stress affects every part of the body, and may play a role in worsening the severity of arthritis. Ginseng is also a powerhouse of antioxidants, which may also protect against arthritic damage. There are several types of ginseng on the market, but I prefer Siberian ginseng, which technically is not ginseng at all, (its a distant cousin) but has many of the same properties, and is therefore used the same way. Regular ginseng can be a potent stimulant, and in some people may cause insomnia.

Although Siberian ginseng produces a nice energy boost, it does not cause sleep problems and, in fact, is used by Asian healers as a treatment for insomnia. All forms of ginseng have a mild estrogenic effect which, in rare cases, may cause side effects such as vaginal bleeding in women. If you are taking ginseng and notice any vaginal bleeding contact your doctor (it could be a sign of another problem) but make sure that he or she knows that you are taking ginseng. Ginseng of any type should not be used by people with high blood pressure or irregular heartbeat.

White willow bark—This herb contains *salicin,* a compound from which aspirin was synthesized. Similar to aspirin, white willow bark has anti-inflammatory properties but, unlike aspirin, contains tannins which are soothing to the stomach. Many of my friends swear by this herb as an arthritis treatment. I personally use it for headaches.

Cartilage Cures

Since all forms of arthritis involve the destruction of cartilage, it makes sense that ingesting forms of cartilage may help relieve symptoms.

Glucosamine sulfate—This natural constituent of cartilage has been shown to produce positive results for sufferers from osteoarthritis; it works to address the underlying cause of the disease by stimulating cartilage repair and is free from side effects. It is sold in natural-food stores.

Shark cartilage—Is it true that sharks don't get arthritis? Maybe. Studies have found that compounds in shark cartilage accelerate the regeneration and repair of cartilage cells. European studies have found that injections of a compound found in shark cartilage are as effective as NSAIDS for treating the symptoms of arthritis.

Chew on a chicken bone—Everyone knows that chicken soup is great for the common cold, but is it also good for arthritis? According to a study by Harvard Medical School researchers, chicken cartilage protein, which is found in chicken bones, can help relieve the symptoms of rheumatoid arthritis. In a clinical study, fifty-nine people with severe rheumatoid arthritis were taken off the drugs they had been using to control their joint pain for the duration of the study.

Each morning twenty-eight patients drank a glass of orange juice containing collagen derived from purified chicken cartilage. The remaining thirty-one volunteers, who served as controls, drank orange juice containing a placebo. After three months, the team noticed a decrease in the number of symptoms and four of the twenty-eight experienced a complete remission of their disease. No improvement was noted in the placebo group.

Antioxidants

Vitamin C—The most famous of the antioxidants, this vitamin is found in citrus fruits; bioflavonoids (related compounds) protect vitamin C by preventing its destruction in the body. A recent review of the physiological action of flavonoids shows a favorable effect on white-blood cells in increasing immune defense, which may account for the resulting anti-inflammatory activity.

Bioflavonoids—These plant compounds are found in lemons, grapes, plums, black currants, grapefruit, apricots, buckwheat, cherries, blackberries, in the white rind of citrus fruits, squash, broccoli, cabbage, parsley, carrots, cucumbers, and rose hips. Bioflavonoids are also available in supplement form.

Vitamin E—This vitamin appears to help alleviate the pain and stiffness of arthritis. A recent study of osteoarthritis showed that vitamin E supplements helped reduce pain, improve mobility, and reduce the need for painkillers.

Minerals

Copper—A long-time folk remedy for arthritis, this mineral is required to convert the body's iron into hemoglobin. It helps to keep bones, blood vessels, and nerves healthy, and the immune system functioning. At one time, copper was considered a possible cause of arthritis because high concentrations of copper were found in the joints of patients with rheumatoid arthritis. It may be, however, that the elevated copper levels could be an attempt on the part of the body to treat itself. In fact, studies have shown that copper included with other anti-inflammatory drugs may help reduce arthritic symptoms. Good food sources include shellfish, whole wheat, beans, nuts, seeds, prunes, and calf and beef liver.

Other Supplements

Omega-3—This refers to the two types of polyunsaturated fatty acids found in fish such as salmon, halibut, albacore tuna, bass, sardines, and mackerel. Omega-3 fatty acids are anti-inflammatory and useful in the treatment of arthritis.

Personal Advice

Lose the excess baggage—The most important dietary recommendation for osteoarthritis sufferers is to achieve normal body weight to lessen the stress on weight-bearing joints. It is critical that the diet be rich in whole natural foods, especially raw fruits and vegetables, because they are a rich source of nutrients critical to joint health, including vitamin C, carotenes, and flavonoids.

Rheumatoid arthritis sufferers may want to eliminate foods from the nightshade family such as potatoes, tomatoes, and eggplant, which are thought to aggravate the condition in some but not all people. Some people find that eliminating all dairy products can also help to relieve symptoms. Smokers take note: Tobacco is a member of the nightshade family!

Retaining flexibility of movement is vital to achieving a better quality of life for arthritis patients. Exercise such as walking, swimming, and stretching are recommended. Because arthritis makes joints stiff and painful, the natural tendency is to minimize movement, which can lead to stiffer joints and more pain since inactivity weakens the muscles that stabilize joints. The secret is to start slowly and never quit.

If you are having a flare-up of symptoms, isometric exercises, which involves tensing muscles but not moving joints, are safe and easy. Also, simple hand exercises such as squeezing a rubber ball, or rotating the foot around a golf ball, can keep joints flexible when more strenuous exercise is not possible.

Earl's Rx

Is your arthritis acting up? These supplements will help soothe those aching joints.

Bromelain: One 500 mg. tablet or capsule twice daily.

Capsaicin : One capsule three times daily.

Evening primrose oil: One capsule three times daily.

Siberian ginseng: One capsule up to twice daily.

White willow bark: One capsule or tablet every three to four hours as needed for pain.

Glucosamine sulfate: One 500 mg. capsule daily.

Omega-3 fatty acids: One 1000 mg. capsule three times daily.

Copper: One (3 mg.) tablet daily.

Grapeseed extract: 30 mg. three times daily.

Asthma

Asthma is the fifth leading cause of death in the United States.

Despite aggressive drug therapy aimed at controlling the disease, asthma and respiratory deaths are rising.

You feel as if an elephant is sitting on your chest; your pulse races as your heart works harder to compensate for the lack of oxygen. Suddenly, you are gasping for air, and panic sets in. I am describing an asthma attack, and as anyone who has suffered from one knows, asthma is not a disease to be dismissed lightly.

Asthma is a respiratory disorder in which the air tubes of the lungs become constricted, impairing breathing. Attacks can be triggered by a variety of factors including allergies, exposure to chemicals, physical exertion, and illnesses which cause inflammation of the lungs (such as the common cold).

In recent years, reported cases of asthma have been on the rise. Why? Although stringent clean-air laws have substantially cut dangerous emissions from industry, incinerators, and automobiles, there is a new and even more dangerous problem—indoor pollution. Since the 1970s, energy-saving new construction has produced almost air-tight buildings, which trap indoor pollutants and can aggravate asthma. In addition, the proliferation of chemically based household products such as air fresheners, synthetic carpets, rugs, and drapes have created indoor environments that experts estimate may be up to *nine times worse* than outdoor air quality even in polluted urban areas.

Diet may also account for the alarming rise in asthma, due to the increase of chemicals in our food, higher amounts of sugar in processed foods, and manmade hydrogenated fats. In addition, since asthma is also a disease of the immune system (allergens can cause the immune system to over-react; producing histamines which generate the production of mucus) the increasing use of antibiotics may be undermining our immune systems.

Finally, there are the drugs themselves which may temporarily relieve symptoms but do nothing to eliminate the disease, resulting in a roller-coaster effect of using drugs, getting temporary relief, suffering another attack, and then increasing the dosage of drugs.

The search for better control of asthma requires expert detective work by the physician to identify any allergies that may be triggering the attack, and willingness from the patient to use whatever techniques are available to build the natural defenses against this insidious disease.

Since asthma is due to the inflammation of the lungs, supplements which prevent or relieve inflammation may help to ward off serious attacks.

Herbs

Licorice—For thousands of years, Chinese healers have used this herb to treat asthma, and it is now available in commercial formulas sold in natural food stores. (Do not use licorice if you have high blood pressure.)

Ginkgo biloba—Ginkgo biloba is a natural anti-inflammatory that can prevent irritation to the breathing passages that may trigger an asthma attack. In addition, ginkgo can improve circulation which, in turn, helps to transport oxygen throughout the body. Very often, due to impaired breathing, asthmatics do not take in enough oxygen, and ginkgo can help them better utilize whatever oxygen they do get by delivering it more efficiently to tissues throughout the body.

Vitamins

Vitamin C—Vitamin C can help suppress the release of histamines, which can aggravate asthma.

Vitamin E—This vitamin is a known anti-inflammatory and may help to prevent attacks.

Herbs

Caffeine—Caffeine is a relative of *theophylline,* a standard asthma drug, which opens the bronchial passages. I usually advise people to avoid caffeine because it is a powerful drug but, in this case, a powerful drug may be just what the doctor ordered. In fact, some asthma sufferers find that when they feel an attack coming on, two strong cups of coffee can often relieve the symptoms.

Parsley tea—A simple tea, made from one cup of hot water poured over a few sprigs of parsley, is a good expectorant and can help clear the lungs.

Onion—Substances found in onion can inhibit the production of compounds that cause the bronchial muscle to spasm. These compounds can also relax the bronchial muscle.

Other Supplements

Quercetin—Quercetin is a member of the bioflavonoid family, compounds found in fruits and vegetables, giving them their distinctive colors. There are more than one thousand different types of bioflavonoids, and scientists are just beginning to unravel their unique and remarkable properties. Studies have shown that quercetin is both an antihistamine, which can block allergic reactions, as well as an anti-inflammatory, which will prevent the breathing passages from becoming irritated.

Bromelain—Found in fresh pineapple, bromelain is a natural digestive aid and also a powerful anti-inflammatory. Bromelain can enhance the action of quercetin by improving its absorption by the body. Bromelain and quercetin are often taken in combination, and may be combined in special herbal and vitamin formulas designed to treat allergy symptoms and asthma.

Personal Advice

Learn to relax—Numerous studies have documented that stress can aggravate or even trigger asthma. Simple relaxation techniques, such as yoga, tai chi, and mediation can help to relieve stress. I also recommend taking extra B vitamins, which are nature's own stress busters.

Clean up your act!—No matter how spic and span you think your house is, it still harbors millions of dust mites, which can trigger an allergic reaction. So can animal dander. Dust mites collect in bedding, carpets, drapes, feather pillows, and blinds. Replace dust catching drapes and blinds with shades, get rid of rugs or at least replace them with those that have a flat nap, and try using nonchemical household cleaning products. I recommend using an air purifier in your home and office.

For allergy sufferers, the bedroom may be the primary battle zone. To minimize the problem, start by encasing the mattress and springs, pillows, and comforters in zippered, allergen-proof covers. Replace wool or feather-filled blankets with washable ones. Wash all bedding once a week in hot water to kill the mites. Get rid of dust-collecting clutter, including stuffed toys and dried flowers.

Eat a low-sugar diet that includes fresh vegetables, magnesium, and omega oils. And read those labels to avoid putting a lot of chemicals into your system that could trigger an allergic reaction.

The foods you eat (or avoid) may help to control asthma symptoms. Obviously, avoid any foods to which are allergic.

Earl's Rx

These supplements should help to keep asthma at bay.

Complex multivitamin with B-complex and digestive enzymes: One tablet with food twice daily. (One in the morning and one in the evening.)

Vitamin B12: One or two 500 mg. to 1000 mg. B12 tablets sublingually (dissolved under the tongue) daily. The sublingual form of this vitamin is better absorbed.

Pantothenic acid: (Part of the B-complex family): Two 500 mg. tablets daily with food.

Licorice: One capsule up to three times daily.

Ginkgo biloba: One (60 mg.) capsule or tablet three times daily.

Bromelain and quercetin combination: Two capsules daily. (If you can't find the combined bromelain/quercetin formula, take two 500 mg. capsules of each daily.)

Vitamin C: Two 500 mg. tablets of calcium ascorbate daily. (Calcium ascorbate is the form of vitamin C that is gentlest on the stomach.)

Vitamin E: 400 IU of vitamin E capsules daily. (Dry form is the best.)

Brittle Nails

Peeling, chipping nails can be a sign of a vitamin deficiency.

They're unsightly, uncomfortable, and very annoying: Brittle, dry, splitting nails are not just a cosmetic problem, but can also be a sign of a nutritional deficiency, illness, or even a fungal infection. Cold weather, stress, a compromised immune system, and lack of certain vitamins can also contribute to this condition.

The run of the mill "brittle-nail syndrome" can often be treated successfully by using a combination of supplements and nail care.

Fungal infections should be treated by a physician or natural healer; they are persistent infections that can cause great discomfort and may spread to other nails. Oral antifungal drugs are typically prescribed to treat the infection, but they are not without side effects, including nausea and upset stomach. In many cases, some tried and true herbal remedies are potent fungus fighters.

Vitamins

Biotin—Biotin, also called *enzyme R* or *vitamin H,* is a member of the B-complex family. It is a water-soluble vitamin, which can be synthesized in the intestines and also can be derived from food. Biotin is necessary for the normal metabolism of fat and protein and for the absorption of vitamin C. This vitamin works with vitamins A, B2, B6, and niacin to maintain healthy skin and nails.

A recent Swiss study involved forty-four patients with thin, brittle nails. Out of thirty-five people who took 300 mcg. biotin supplements daily, 63 percent showed clinical improvement in their nails, with increased thickness of the nails and less splitting.

Although no side effects from this high dose have been reported, I recommend that biotin be taken for three months, stopped for one month, and then continued. I believe that this system will prevent blood levels of biotin from becoming too high. Good food sources include fruit, nuts, brewer's yeast, beef liver, peanut butter, cauliflower, egg yolk, and whole-grain foods.

Minerals

Calcium—If your nails are brittle and constantly dry, splitting, chipping, and peeling, include more calcium-rich foods in your diet. These include broccoli, collard greens, low-fat dairy products, and calcium-fortified juices. Calcium is also available as a supplement.

Herbs

Silica—Also known as *horsetail,* this herb has been used by natural healers in Europe and China for many years. It is rich in nutrients, including silicon. Silica facilitates the absorption of calcium by the body; calcium nourishes nails in addition to skin, hair, bones, and the body's connective tissue.

Almond oil—Try soaking fingertips in warm almond oil for fifteen minutes, then rub oil into cuticles, hands, and feet. The oil will nourish the nails, making them less dry and brittle—and it leaves the skin feeling soft and smooth. (Warm olive oil also works well.)

Tea tree oil—Candida (a genus of yeast fungi) of the nails is the most frequent cause of nail disease and brittle nails. Standard therapy includes topical antifungals and oral medications. Unfortunately, fungal infections don't always respond to standard treatment, and the rate of recurrence is very high.

Tea tree, an herb long used in the tropics to treat yeast and fungal infections, appears to help control fungal infections of the nail when applied directly. A recent study compared the results of treatments with standard therapy to that of 100 percent tea-tree oil for the treatment of fungal infections of the nails. One-hundred-seventeen patients took part in a study for six months. Half received standard antifungal treatment and half had the tea-oil solution applied to the infected nails. Debridement (surgical removal of infected nail tissue and foreign matter) was performed at the beginning of treatment and again in the first, third, and sixth month of treatment.

Results after six months of treatment indicate that topical application of tea oil, together with debridement, provided improvement in both the appearance of the nail and the symptoms of the infection and worked better than debridement alone.

Nail Strengtheners

Glucosamine sulfate—Glucosamine sulfate helps strengthen collagen, which is essential for the growth of skin and nails.

Personal Advice

Take good care of your nails! A few simple measures can go a long way in keeping them healthy. Nail polish helps protect the nail bed and helps to slow down loss of moisture in nails, but use only formaldehyde- and acetone-free remover. (Acetone can dry out nails.)

Acrylic nails are acceptable, but you might consider doing a skin test before use to be sure you are not allergic to acrylic. Acrylic nails must be removed every three months to give nails time to breath. If acrylic nails are left on indefinitely, moisture will gather under the nail plate, which can result in separation of the nail as well as fungal infections.

In addition to tea-tree oil, any moisturizer will help nails become less brittle, especially during the winter. Remove nail polish, soak fingertips in warm water for about ten minutes, then apply moisturizer.

Wear gloves while doing housework, especially when using abrasive cleaning agents. And please don't use your nails as tools.

Earl's Rx

For strong nails, try the following.

Biotin: One tablet (300 mcg.) up to three times daily.

Calcium and vitamin D: One tablet or capsule, 1200 mg. calcium with 400 IU Vitamin D daily.

Nail-Strengthening Formula : This special combination of supplements is packaged in capsule form and is designed to help strengthen nails, skin, and hair. Several different versions of this formula are sold in natural-food stores, but they are all basically the same and will do an equally good job.

The combination includes glucosamine sulfate (500 mg.), silica, sulfur, SOD (super oxide dismutase), essential fatty acids, and zinc.

Bruises

Think P for pineapple and Vitamin P for bioflavonoids.

They're ugly and they can be quite painful. A bruise or *contusion*, is an area of skin discoloration caused by the rupture of underlying vessels following injury. A bruise usually starts out a reddish color, gradually becomes bluish, then greenish yellow as the hemoglobin in the tissues breaks down chemically and is absorbed by the body.

You can expect a bruise to follow trauma such as a blow or fall—that's only natural and, after a few days, the body will heal itself. However, if bruising appears frequently and with no apparent cause, it is advisable to see a physician, as frequent bruising can be an indication of a more serious problem.

Most bruises need no treatment, but this is an area where common sense is the first line of defense. Naturally, if a trauma caused bleeding or the skin is scraped, the area needs to be gently cleaned and an antibacterial ointment or cream should be applied.

If the injury causes swelling, ice applied to the damaged area decreases the bleeding from the torn blood vessels and limits swelling. Since swelling slows the healing process, wrapping the area compresses the injured part and limits the build-up of fluids. Finally, elevating the injured part above the level of the heart makes use of gravity to help drain fluids out of the injured area. Ice can be used in fifteen-minute intervals for 20 minutes at a time a few times daily to help improve circulation. Heat increases the flow of nutrients and removes the damaged tissues, thus stimulating healing. Wait a few days after the injury, until the acute inflammation has subsided, before using heat.

Herbs

Herbal remedies are time-honored ways to decrease inflammation and promote healing.

Arnica—The flower and root of arnica have been used by natural healers for generations as pain relievers. Rubbed on the skin, it is great for healing wounds, bruises, or other skin irritations. Arnica should not be taken internally unless it is in the much weakened homeopathic form (Dose:10–30x). Many doctors are now prescribing homeopathic arnica to their patients before surgery to speed healing and prevent bruising.

Herbal ointments—Ointments made with eucalyptus oil, salicylates, and menthol contain natural anesthetics and will help relieve pain. Liniments contain counterirritants and help decrease pain and increase circulation to the injury by irritating the skin over it. Typical counterirritants include *methyl salicylate* (oil of wintergreen) and *camphor.*

Comfrey—If the bruise is still a problem after a few days, an ointment made with comfrey-root extract can be applied locally. Comfrey contains *allatoin,* a substance that is absorbed through the skin and helps stimulate the growth of new cells. (Comfrey should not be used internally.)

Bromelain—This enzyme, which is found in pineapple, has been shown to facilitate repair of damaged tissues and lessen inflammation. Bromelain breaks down quickly when it is exposed to fresh air so, for best results, get a fresh pineapple and eat it right away. Some researchers even advise runners to eat fresh pineapple before a race to prevent bruising! Bromelain tablets are also available.

Vitamins

Bioflavonoids—The *bioflavonoids,* a group of substances related to vitamin C, can speed the healing of bruises. A report in *Medical Times* stated that athletes taking citrus bioflavonoids and vitamin C healed twice as fast as athletes who took either vitamin C alone or no supplements. Another study found that injured football players who took 200 to 600 mg. daily of citrus bioflavonoids returned to the game more quickly than those not taking supplements.

Kiwifruit, currants, oranges, apples, cranberries, blueberries, papaya, strawberries, avocados, pineapples, blackberries, grapes, figs, bananas, and grapefruits blended together will produce a powerhouse of vitamin C and citrus bioflavonoids.

Personal Advice

Once again, common sense should prevail in the event of an injury. If the trauma causes severe pain, if the injury is to a joint or its ligaments, if there is numbness or loss of function (for instance, if you can't move fingers or toes), or if you suspect a fracture, don't self-treat. See a doctor.

If you end up with a lot of bruises after certain activities, such as aerobics, running, or tennis, it might be wise to re-evaluate your skills, equipment, and the area where the activity takes place.

Finally, eat plenty of fresh fruit and vegetables, get enough sleep, and exercise on a regular basis; a healthy body is less likely to bruise easily.

Earl's Rx

If you bruise easily, try the following.

Special bruise-busting formula: This combination of supplements designed to promote bruise healing is sold in many natural-food stores. Look for C-complex with bioflavonoids, including hesperidin and bromelain. Take 1000–4000 mg. daily until the bruises are healed.

In addition, add 500 mg. of rutin, another bioflavonoid, to the regimen until the bruises are healed.

Cancer

Cancer is the second most common cause of death in the United States.

According to the National Cancer Institute, about half of all cancers may be preventable through changes in diet and lifestyles.

There are many different types of cancer but, basically, all forms of cancer involve the abnormal growth of cells. In order to understand what cancer is, and why it is such a threat, I want you to think of your body as a giant factory involving literally billions of workers: in this case, the workers are individual cells. Cells are the workhorses of the body; they are involved in virtually every bodily function. Throughout our lives, cells are continually growing, reproducing, transforming ingested food into energy, and repairing damage to the organs and tissues of the body. At the core of this activity is the death and regeneration of millions of cells every day. Normal cells multiply and differentiate into specialized individual types that are programmed to perform specific tasks within a particular bodily system. For example, the cells of the lung have a particular function involved in breathing, while the cells of the heart are designed to keep that vital organ continuously beating. Within these systems the cells "mind their own business," with each cell tending to its designated place, size, and responsibility. The cancer process begins when an errant cell mutates, that is, undergoes a change, and begins to multiply wildly. These "bad" cells forget what they were designed to do and, as they grow, invade neighboring groups of cells, robbing them of precious nutrients. If these abnormal cells are allowed to grow unfettered, they can eventually kill off the healthy cells, destroying important organ systems. To go back to the analogy of the giant factory, it is as if one group of workers on an assembly line were to invade other parts of the assembly line, preventing the other vital workers from performing their jobs. In real life, the assembly line would eventually shut down and would no longer able be able to function. In your body, as cancer spreads, it can invade various organ systems, making it impossible for your body to function normally.

Why and how these cancer cells run amok is the $64,000 question; there are many theories as to why cells turn malignant, but few concrete answers. We do know that some types of cancer are hereditary. For example, in women, a particular gene has been identified with an increased risk of breast cancer, and that same gene has been implicated with prostate cancer in men. The majority of cancer cases, however, are not believed to be genetic. In fact, the National Cancer Institute estimates that at least half of all cases of cancer are caused by environmental factors such as smoking, excessive drinking, diet, and lifestyle. What is particularly intriguing is the fact that within the past five years, there has been a tremendous amount of research devoted to the role that various foods and supplements may play in helping to keep cancer at bay.

Food as medicine—There is exciting new evidence that vitamins, minerals, and naturally occurring compounds in fruits and vegetables called *phytochemicals* may help to prevent many different diseases, including various forms of cancer. (For more information, I refer you to *Earl Mindell's Food as Medicine*, Fireside, 1994.) For example, many foods contain natural antioxidants which may help to protect against cancer-causing elements in our environment that can promote the formation of free radicals in the body. As I have discussed earlier, free radicals are unstable oxygen atoms that bind readily with other atoms. When free radicals bind with other atoms, they emit energy which can damage healthy cells and cause them to mutate. There are two kinds of antioxidants; some intervene at various stages to prevent the formation of free radicals, and others called *free radical scavengers* mop up whatever free radicals are circulating throughout the body before they can cause damage. Tobacco smoke, pollutants, solvents, and pesticides are all believed to promote the formation of damaging free radicals. The army of antioxidants include familiar names such as vitamin C, vitamin E, selenium, zinc, and copper, and some exotic sounding compounds such as *lycopene* and *lutein*, both members of the carotenoid family, a group of more than 600 compounds naturally occurring in fruits and vegetables. (I will discuss antioxidants as they pertain to particular cancers later.) In order to get enough natural antioxidants, you must eat at least five servings of fruits and vegetables throughout the day. (For fruits, one serving is defined as one medium fruit or 6 ounces of fresh fruit juice. For vegetables, one serving is defined as one cup raw, leafy vegetables or 6 ounces of vegetable juice.) Few Americans actually do eat enough fruits and vegetables and, frankly, I am skeptical that it is actually possible to get enough antioxidants through diet alone. Fortunately, many antioxidants found in food are now available in supplement form. I believe that everyone should take a broad-spectrum vitamin/mineral supplement with antioxidants, including alpha and beta carotene, vitamins C, E, selenium, and *glutathione,* an amino acid. In addition, depending on your age, sex, personal medical history, and genetics you may want to add particular supplements that may help prevent specific types of cancer.

Prostate Cancer

P rostate cancer is the second most common cancer in men (skin cancer is number one), and is of great concern because it appears to be increasing. The prostate is a small, walnut-sized gland between the bladder and penis, above the rectum. (For general information on prostate health, see page 234.) More than two hundred thousand men are diagnosed with prostate cancer each year, and it is responsible for close to forty thousand deaths annually.

The risk of developing prostate cancer greatly increases with age. It rarely occurs in men younger than fifty and the average age of onset is seventy-two. The cause of prostate cancer is unknown, but continuing research has uncovered an intriguing connection between diet and prostate cancer. A study published in the *Journal of the National Cancer Institute* (1993), reported the result of research that measured the relationship between high-fat diets and prostate cancer. Total saturated-fat consumption was found to be directly related to the risk of advanced prostate cancer. This association was due primarily to animal fat. Interestingly, red meat, which is high in saturated fat, represented the food group with the strongest positive association with advanced cancer. Fat from dairy products, with the exception of butter, or fish was unrelated to risk. The results support the hypothesis that animal fat, especially fat from red meat, is associated with an elevated risk of advanced prostate cancer.

Soy—Cutting back on red meat may be one way to reduce the risk of developing prostate cancer, and eating soy foods is another. American men are *five times* more likely to die of prostate cancer than are native Japanese men, but when they move to the United States, Japanese men lose their advantage within a generation. The typical Japanese diet includes 3–4 ounces of soy foods daily, including tofu, soy milk, and soy beans. This fact has led many researchers to suspect that the traditional Japanese diet may somehow protect against prostate cancer and, more specifically, that soy foods, which dominate Japanese cuisine, may be the protective factor.

Isoflavones—Soy is a rich source of phytochemicals called *isoflavones,* hormonelike compounds that mimic the action of hormones in the human body but are far weaker. Researchers believe that isoflavones may inhibit the growth of particular types of tumors that are hormone dependent, that is, whose growth is stimulated by hormones that occur naturally in the body. The theory is that these plant hormones bind to receptors on hormone-dependent tumors that would normally be occupied by the body's own more potent hormones that would trigger growth. These plant hormones, however, have just the opposite effect on tumors, and can prevent growth.

Soy is the only known source of *genistein,* an isoflavone that has been shown in laboratory experiments to inhibit enzymes that trigger the growth of prostate tumor cells. Interestingly, studies in Japan revealed that although Japanese men develop prostate cancers as often as American men, the cancers in the Japanese men develop very slowly, with many men never showing the clinical signs of the disease. Researchers found that genistein blocked the enzymes that triggered cell growth, and suspect that it may slow down the disease to the point that it never becomes a problem. In addition, genistein can help promote cell differentiation in cancerous cells, that is, it can help specialized cells "remember" their particular job in the body. This is good because undifferentiated cells are very resistant to cancer therapies. In yet another study, an international group of researchers at Children's University Hospital in Heidelberg found yet another potential mechanism by which genistein can prevent the spread of cancer. Angiogenesis is the generation of new capillaries or small blood vessels, a process that should only occur under certain conditions, such as wound healing or pregnancy, but can be triggered by tumors, which need new capillaries to deliver nourishment in order to grow. Genistein was shown to block this process in laboratory studies. Genistein is available in supplement form.

Soy foods also contain other anticancer compounds that may play a role in the prevention of all types of cancer including prostate cancer.

Daidzein— Daidzein is another isoflavone found in soy. It has been shown in recent laboratory studies to inhibit the growth of cancer cells and promote cell differentiation in animals.

Protease inhibitors—You may have heard a great deal recently about compounds called *protease inhibitors,* because they are being touted as the hot new treatment for AIDS. Protease inhibitors are compounds that block the growth of particular cells by inhibiting the action of proteases, enzymes that promote tumor growth. (In AIDS patients, protease inhibitors appear to thwart the replication of HIV, the virus that causes AIDS.) According to researchers at the University of Pennsylvania School of Medicine, soy contains a unique protease inhibitor that shows promise of being a potent anticarcinogen that may prevent or inhibit the growth a wide range of cancers, including prostate cancer.

Lycopene—Carotenoids are the compounds in fruits and vegetables that give them color, and many are believed to have anticancer properties. For example, one member of the carotenoid family, *lycopene,* may help prevent prostate cancer. Lycopene is found in many fruits and vegetables, with tomatoes, watermelon, and palm oil being particularly rich sources. It is now available as a supplement. Recently, Harvard Universit researchers reported that men who eat at least ten servings a week of tomato-based foods sharply reduce their risk of developing prostate cancer, and they speculated that lycopene could be the protective factor. In another study, German researchers have recently shown that lycopene can reduce free-radical damage in cells exposed to chemicals that promote the formation of free radicals.

Lutein—Lutein is another member of the carotenoid family with potent antioxidant properties. Lutein is abundant in green vegetables such as kale, spinach, and broccoli. Since most men do not eat these foods routinely, I recommend taking a lutein supplement.

Earl's Rx

Soy: Take one scoop of soy powdered beverage (be sure it contains isoflavones, genistein, and daidzen) and blend into 8 ounces of low-fat or no-fat soy milk. (Vanilla flavored is my favorite!) Add a few ice cubes and mix in blender. Drink daily as a meal or between-meals snack.

Antioxidant formula for prostate health: All men should take a good antioxidant formula designed specifically for prostate health. There are several excellent combination formulas sold at natural food stores. Select one that includes genistein, daidzein, lycopene, and lutein. Take one capsule up to three times daily with food.

Breast Cancer

B reast cancer is the second leading cause of cancer deaths among women (lung cancer is number one). More than 200,000 are diagnosed with this disease each year, and more than 46,000 women die of it.

As I mentioned earlier, a small number of breast cancer cases (roughly 6 percent) have been linked to a particular gene, but in most cases, we simply do not know what causes breast cancer. The relationship between diet and breast cancer has been closely scrutinized. Similar to prostate cancer, breast cancer is more common in western countries and relatively rare in Asia and Africa. Many researchers strongly suspect that diet, in particular the high-fat diet typical of the west, is at least a contributing factor in the high rate of breast cancer in countries such as the United States. Americans consume about 36 percent of their daily caloric intake in fat, much of it in the form of saturated fat from meat and dairy products. In comparison, Asians consume under 15 percent of their daily calories in fat, and much of that in the form of polyunsaturated or vegetable fat. A handful of studies have shown a connection between a high-fat diet and midline obesity (bulging abdomen), which we know is a risk factor for breast cancer. At least one other study has shown a direct correlation between fat intake and the recurrence of cancer in women who had been previously diagnosed with breast cancer. Even though studies that have attempted to link fat intake to breast cancer have been inconclusive, given that a high-fat diet is a risk factor for heart disease and other forms of cancer, in particular colon cancer, it makes sense to limit your fat intake to under 20 percent of total calories.

Fat may only be part of the story; fiber intake appears to be equally important. For example, Finnish women eat a diet that is even higher in fat than American women, yet their mortality rate for breast cancer is considerably lower. Unlike American women, however, Finnish women eat a diet that is very high in fiber, which researchers believe may protect against breast cancer, and may actually counteract the damaging effect of a high-fat diet. Fiber helps to move food through the gut more rapidly, thus helping the body rid itself of toxins (such as insecticides and other chemicals) more rapidly before they can do harm. In addition, some studies have shown that certain forms of fiber, such as wheat fiber, can help to reduce the level of certain forms of potent estrogens that may trigger the growth of breast tumors.

Soy—Like prostate cancer, at least 75 percent of all breast cancers are *hormone dependent,* which means that they can be stimulated to grow by estrogen. In fact, some but not all studies have shown that women who develop breast cancer have higher than normal levels of a particularly potent form of estrogen. Similar to the role they play in prostate tumors, isoflavones in soy can bind to estrogen receptors in the breast and actually inhibit the growth of tumors. In addition, studies have suggested that genistein may be effective against tumors that are not estrogen sensitive. In test tube studies at the University of Alabama, researchers found that genistein stopped the growth of nonestrogen-sensitive breast cancer cells, and that the presence of an estrogen receptor is not necessary for isoflavones to inhibit tumor growth. This suggests that the protective effect of isoflavones may not be due to their effect on hormones, but on the ability of genistein to block cell growth. It is interesting to note that American women are four times more likely to die from breast cancer than Japanese women, and the one consistent difference between the two groups appears to be the intake of soy foods. Experts recommend that women consume at least 40 mg. of isoflavones daily. To achieve this level, you need to drink 1 cup of soy milk daily or eat about 3–4 ounces of tofu. If you do not eat soy foods on a regular basis, powdered soy protein beverages that are rich in isoflavones and prepared soy shakes are available at natural-food stores or by mail order.

Flax—Thousands of years ago, flaxseed was a normal part of the human diet but today it is primarily used to make fabric. Flaxseed is rich in *lignans,* compounds that are similar to natural estrogens produced by the body. Lignans are believed to deactivate potent estrogens that can trigger the growth of tumors. Flaxseed oil is sold in capsule or liquid form at natural-food stores. Keep the oil refrigerated.

Selenium—In a study reported in *The European Journal of Cancer Prevention* (1991), women who consumed the highest levels of the mineral selenium had the lowest rate of death from breast cancer. This makes good sense, as we know that selenium is a potent antioxidant that can protect against many different forms of cancer. Good food sources of selenium include garlic, onions, fish, shellfish, red grapes, broccoli, whole wheat and grains, eggs, Brazil nuts, and chicken. Selenium is also available in supplement form.

Limonene—Animal studies have shown that this compound found in the essential oils of citrus fruits and lemon grass can inhibit the growth of breast tumors. Recently, London's Charing Cross Hospital began a trial of limonene in women to see if it might be useful as a treatment for breast cancer. A good source of limonene is the soft white pulp surrounding citrus fruit; it is also available in supplement form.

Melatonin—An interesting research finding regarding breast-cancer risk implies that women exposed to low-frequency electromagnetic fields are more at risk of breast cancer, because exposure to such fields can reduce the pineal gland's nighttime production of an anticancer hormone called *melatonin*. Reduced concentrations of melatonin in the blood spur the growth of breast-cancer cells, suggest researchers at the Pacific Northwest laboratory in Richland, Washington. Studies are continuing to ascertain whether exposure to household appliances such as microwave ovens, televisions, and hair dryers can increase the risk of breast and other cancers. Melatonin is available in capsules and tablets.

Earl's Rx

Soy shake: Take one scoop of soy powdered beverage (be sure it contains isoflavones, genistein, and daidzen) and blend into 8 ounces of low-fat or no-fat soy milk. Add a few ice cubes and mix in blender. Drink daily.

Flax seed oil: One tablespoon of oil or three capsules daily. (Special flaxseed products are sold in natural-food stores.) Only use products that contain stabilized flaxseed, as ordinary flaxseed can become rancid very quickly.

Selenium: One 100 mcg. tablet or capsule daily with food.

Melatonin: Take 1 mg. sublingual capsule (dissolves under the tongue for better absorption) 5–15 minutes before bedtime. (Melatonin will make you very drowsy; do not drive after taking it.)

Skin Cancer

Skin cancer is the most common cancer among men and is fast becoming a major threat for both sexes. Men on average spend more than twice as much time in the sun as do women, and are much more likely to die from *melanoma,* the most lethal form of this disease than are women. In fact, the rate of melanoma among both men and women has increased exponentially in recent years, and there is no dispute as to the reason why: Nearly everyone agrees that overexposure to sunlight can cause skin cancer.

It is widely believed that the ultraviolet rays in sunlight can increase the production of free radicals, which can in turn destroy healthy cells and turn them cancerous. Sunscreens can help to filter out damaging UVA and UVB rays, and can prevent sunburns, but many researchers believe that any sign of skin tanning is evidence of skin damage, and that exposure to sun should be severely limited.

Antioxidants—Studies also suggest that antioxidants, either from food or in supplement form, can reduce the risk of skin cancer. For example, one recent Australian study showed a significant inverse relationship between the risk of skin cancer and consumption of vegetables such as Swiss chard, pumpkin, cabbage, Brussels sprouts, and broccoli. These foods contain high levels of several different types of carotenoids including alphacarotene, betacarotene, and vitamin C, which are known antioxidants.

In addition, researchers at the Department of Nutrition Sciences, University of Alabama at Birmingham, conducted laboratory tests to determine the effect of antioxidant nutrients on skin cancers. Results indicate that increased oral doses of vitamin E and glutathione reduced the risk of skin cancers in rats.

Another potent broad-spectrum antioxidant is grapeseed extract, which contains compounds called *proanthrocyanodins.* Proanthrocyanodins are potent antioxidants, and are present in wine and grape juice.

Cut the fat—A high-fat diet may also play a role in increasing the risk of skin cancer. That's the theory advanced by researchers at the Veterans Affairs Medical Center in Houston, Texas, who say a low-fat diet reduces the risk of lesions that lead to the most common cancer among white men in the United States.

Researchers at the Verteran's Affairs Medical Center randomly assigned seventy-six patients who had been diagnosed with non-melanoma-type skin cancer (which is more common than melanoma) to one of two groups. Members in one group were put on a low-fat diet (20 percent of calories from fat), the other group continued to eat their usual diet (40 percent of calories from fat). After two years, each low-fat group member averaged three precancerous lesions (called *actinic ker-*

atoses) a month. The members of the higher-fat–consuming group averaged ten lesions. Why and how fat stimulates tumor growth is not fully understood; what is becoming apparent however is that a diet high in fat can increase the risk of many different types of cancers.

Personal advice—Always use an effective sunblock (SPF factor of at least fifteen) when you are out in the sun.

Earl's Rx

Antioxidant complex formula: To protect against skin cancer, I recommend a comprehensive antioxidant formula containing alpha and betacarotene, vitamin C, vitamin E, selenium, grapeseed extract, and green-tea extract.

Stomach Cancer

In the U.S., about 25,000 cases of stomach cancer are diagnosed each year, and researchers believe that a combination of dietary therapy and supplements may help to cut the risk of developing this type of cancer.

The widespread use of refrigeration in the U.S. has greatly reduced the number of cases of stomach cancer in the western world. This is because certain naturally occurring compounds found in food can spoil and turn carcinogenic if food is not properly refrigerated. Stomach cancer, however, is still fairly common in China, where refrigeration is not as prevalent, particularly in small rural villages. There is evidence, however, that vitamins, particularly antioxidants, can help reduce the risk of stomach cancer.

Antioxidants—A combined effort by American and Chinese investigators researched the effect of combined vitamin supplements on cancer (particularly esophageal and stomach cancer) on approximately thirty-thousand residents of a rural village in China. After about five years, the researchers discovered that people taking a specific antioxidant vitamin-mineral combination (beta carotene, vitamin E, and selenium) experienced a statistically significant drop in their death rate from all causes, not just cancer. Those taking the combined supplement showed a thirteen-percent drop in deaths from all types of cancer and a twenty-one percent decline in stomach cancer deaths.

Nitrosamine blockers—Certain food additives are also implicated as a causative factor in stomach cancer. For example, *nitrites*, an additive used to cure meats such as bacon and hot dogs, combine with amino acids in the stomach and form compounds called *nitrosamines*, which are highly carcinogenic. Nitrosamines can destroy DNA and lead to cancerous changes in cells.

There are many other common foods consumed by Americans that can reduce the damage of nitrosamines. Two years ago, Cornell University food scientists published data showing that eating green peppers, pineapples, carrots, strawberries, and, especially, tomatoes, can suppress the formation of nitrosamines in humans. Although it is well-known that these foods contain a lot of vitamin C, which in itself can sidetrack the formation of nitrosamines, researchers set out to find what they felt was an even more potent nitrosamine blocker than could be accounted for by vitamin C alone.

Cornell researchers identified two new nitrosamine blockers—*p-coumaric* and *chlorogenic acids*, which provide about forty percent of tomato's nitrosamine-inhibiting activity.

Garlic—Garlic is another potent nitrosamine buster. In a study at the Beijing Institute for Cancer Research, interviews with 564 patients with stomach cancer and 1,131 cancer-free residents in an area of China where stomach cancer rates are high revealed a significant reduction in stomach-cancer risk with increased consumption of allium vegetables. Allium vegetables are any of various plants characterized by their pungent odor, including onions, leeks, chives, garlic, and shallots.

The ability of garlic to inhibit the formation of nitrosamines was corroborated in a Pennsylvania State University research study conducted on rats, which showed that the addition of garlic powder to their diet produced a significant decrease in the development of cancers.

Green tea—A reduced risk of stomach cancers was also found in Japan among heavy tea drinkers. Several studies comparing the diets of those diagnosed cases of stomach cancer versus those who were cancer free showed that people who drank green tea more frequently or in larger quantities tended to have a lower risk of stomach cancer. Researchers speculate that compounds in green tea must have a protective effect against nitrosamines.

Earl's Rx

Antioxidant complex formula: I recommend an antioxidant complex formula including alpha and betacarotene, vitamin C, vitamin E, and selenium. Take two capsules daily with food.

Green tea: Drink 2–3 cups of green tea daily or take a supplement of green-tea extract (no caffeine) twice or three times daily.

Garlic: One 500 mg. raw, aged, odorless garlic tablet or capsule daily.

Oral Cancer

About seventy-five percent of all oral cancers are caused by excessive alcohol intake, chewing tobacco, and smoking. Clearly, simply eliminating these activities could go a long way in reducing the risk of this type of cancer. However, recent research reveals that vitamins and certain phytochemicals may also help.

Vitamin E—A study by the National Cancer Institute, Division of Cancer Etiology in Bethesda, Maryland, suggests that vitamin E may slash the risk of oral cancers by half. In this study, researchers compared the vitamin intake of 1,100 people with oral cancer to nearly 1,300 cancer-free people. One striking fact emerged from this study: Those who took vitamin E supplements showed a substantially lower risk of developing oral or throat cancers. Since vitamin E levels in foods are low, it may make sense to add a vitamin E supplement to your daily regimen.

Although the precise mechanism of how vitamin E works as a cancer protector is not fully understood, researchers attribute it to its ability to fend off unstable harmful molecules called free radicals, and they suspect it may also work by enhancing immune function, which would strengthen the body's ability to weed out cancerous cells.

Betacarotene—There is also some evidence that betacarotene, which is found naturally in many green leafy vegetables and carrots, may deter mouth cancer. A preliminary study treated people with precancerous oral lesions with 60 mg. of beta carotene a day for six months. (This would equal about four to five carrots a day.) Test results showed an impressive fifty-percent reduction in the number of lesions.

Green tea—Drinking green tea has also been linked to a reduced risk of oral cancer in humans, particularly cancer of the esophagus. A study reported in the *Journal of the National Cancer Institute* (June, 1994), compared 900 middle-aged Chinese men and women with esophageal cancer to over 1,500 cancer-free men and women. Among nonsmokers who did not drink alcohol, drinking green tea cut the risk for esophageal cancer by as much as sixty percent. Researchers attribute green tea's anticancer properties to its antioxidant components called *polyphenols*.

Spirulina—The blue-green microalgae spirulina sold in natural food stores in America, have been found to be a rich natural source of proteins, carotenoids, and other micronutrients. Experimental studies in animal models have demonstrated an inhibitory effect of Spirulina algae on oral cancers.

A study reported in *Nutrition and Cancer* (1995) that was conducted among tobacco chewers in India reported a complete regression of precancerous mouth lesions in 45 percent of subjects who were given extracts of spirulina for twelve months. This was the first human study using spirulina as a cancer therapy, and undoubtedly, more studies will follow.

Earl's Rx

Vitamin E: Two (400 IU) capsules daily with food; dry form preferred because it is better absorbed.

Betacarotene: One 5000–10,000 IU capsule daily.

Green tea: Drink one to three cups of green tea daily, or take one to three green-tea extract tablets daily.

Spirulina: One or two tablets daily one half hour before eating.

Cervical Cancer

E ach year, six thousand American women die of cervical cancer. The right supplements may help to dramatically reduce the risk of getting this form of cancer.

Folic acids—A new study from the University of Alabama at Birmingham appears to have uncovered a connection between folic-acid (the B vitamin called *folacin*) deficiency and the risk of developing cervical cancer. In one study reported in *The Journal of the American Medical Association* (1992), 726 women were screened for cervical cancer. Multiple factors were found to increase the risk of cervical cancer risk, including early age at first intercourse, exposure to many different sexual partners, and, possibly, cigarette smoking.

The most significant risk factor for cervical cancer was infection with the human papilomavirus (HPV), which can cause genital warts and cervical dysplasia, abnormal cell growth which can later lead to cancer. Surprisingly, women with HPV who had high blood levels of folic acid had a much lower rate of cervical dysplasia than women with low levels of folic acid. No link was discovered between any other vitamin and cervical cancer. Researchers speculate that folic acid must somehow have a protective effect against the HPV virus. Citrus fruits and tomatoes, grains, yeast, liver, and leafy green vegetables are excellent sources of folic acid, which is also available in supplement form.

Lycopene—Lycopene, a carotenoid compound known to be a free-radical–damage fighter, also appears to protect against cervical cancer. One recent study, reported in the *International Journal of Cancer*, looked at the dietary habits and blood carotenoid levels of 102 women with cervical dysplasia and an equal number of cancer-free women. The women whose intake of lycopene-rich foods was the highest had a substantially lower risk of cervical dysplasia than women with the lowest intake of lycopene. The difference between low and high intake was one tomato a day. Even processed tomato sauce and tomato paste contain high amounts of the carotenoid. Ruby-red grapefruit and sweet red peppers are also good sources of lycopene. Lycopene is also available in supplement form.

Smokers beware: A study was conducted by researchers at the Departments of Nutrition Sciences and Epidemiology at the University of Alabama at Birmingham, the Arkansas Cancer Research Center, Little Rock, and the Medical Nutritional Product R & D, Columbus, Ohio, to determine the effects of smoking on folic acid and vitamin B-12 concentrations in the circulation and in tissues directly exposed to cigarette smoke.

The results showed that smoking had a negative effect on the ability of the body to store, utilize, and benefit from vitamin B-12, and those with higher levels of B-12 showed less risk of developing cervical cancers. Smokers need more folate and more B-12 intake than those who do not smoke. Better yet, don't smoke!

Earl's Rx

Folic acid: Take one 800 mcg. capsule or tablet daily.

Lycopene: Take one 10 mg. tablet or capsule daily.

Lung Cancer

While breast cancer is primarily a woman's disease, lung cancer has long been regarded as a man's disease. That's because it is the number-one cancer killer of men and, until recently, has not been considered a major threat to women. In 1994, however, researchers at the Anderson Cancer Center in Houston made the startling announcement that an estimated 56,000 women would die of lung cancer that year, giving it the dubious distinction of being the number-one cancer killer of women. About 85 percent of all cases of lung cancer are caused by smoking, a habit that women took up in great numbers after World War II. Sadly, the effects of decades of smoking are now exacting a steep toll on women.

Cigarette smoke contains known carcinogens that promote the formation of free radicals, which can injure healthy tissue. Smoking is not only dangerous to the smoker, but it is also harmful to people who must inhale second-hand smoke.

The best way to prevent lung cancer is not to smoke, and not to breath in smoke. Keep in mind that exposure to smoke is just one of several pollutants that we breath in daily. Depending on where you live, the air is filled with smog, exhaust from automobiles and buses, and ozone, which can also promote the formation of free radicals within our bodies. It is essential that we fortify ourselves against free radical attack by taking enough antioxidants.

Vitamin E—Vitamin E is an important weapon in the fight to nullify the effects of these free radicals on delicate lung tissue, which, in turn, helps protect us against lung cancer. Vitamin E is a potent antioxidant, and frankly, I don't know any serious researcher in the field of aging who is not taking a vitamin E supplement.

Carotenoids—Research has shown that low intake of vegetables, fruits, and carotenoids is consistently associated with increased risk of lung cancer. Carotenoids are found primarily in fruits and vegetables, and from the retinol in dairy products, eggs, liver, and fortified cereals.

As previously discussed in this chapter, green tea appears to have an inhibitory effect on cancer-causing agents in the body. The Japanese preference for green tea may explain why Japanese men smoke more than American men, but still have lower rates of lung cancer. Researchers found that consumption of green tea cut the lung-cancer rate by 45 percent in laboratory mice. However, don't think that lighting up a cigarette and then drinking a cup of tea is going to protect you from lung cancer, because while researchers might think drinking green tea may be one of the most practical cancer preventatives, this theory is still just a theory. It is irrefutable that if you stop smoking altogether, you definitely increase your chances of remaining lung-cancer free.

The fat factor—While smoking is known to cause cancer, we still don't know why almost 23,000 nonsmokers die from lung cancer every year in the United States. That number represents about fifteen percent of all lung-cancer deaths.

In an article reported in the *Journal of the National Cancer Institute* (1994), epidemiologists at the Yale University School of Medicine studied the relationship between diet and the risk of lung cancer among nonsmokers. The team recruited 826 men and women; half had lung cancer, and the other half served as controls. All participants in the study were either nonsmokers or had quit smoking at least a decade prior to the study.

Researchers asked the volunteers to estimate their usual consumption of twenty-six different food items. A statistical analysis showed that consumption of raw vegetables and fresh fruits significantly reduced a nonsmoker's chance of developing lung cancer. Estimates show that nonsmokers can reduce their lung cancer risk by an astonishing forty percent by simply adding one-and-a-half servings of such fruits or vegetables to their daily diets.

Selenium—Yet another study linking lung-cancer risk to diet involved more than 120,000 Dutch men and women aged fifty-five to sixty-nine. Patients were tested for blood levels of various vitamins, minerals, and carotenes. People with high levels of selenium, another important antioxidant, were found to have a lower risk of lung cancer. Selenium is involved in the production of glutathione peroxidase, an enzyme that protects cells against oxidative damage.

Earl's Rx

Vitamin E: Up to two 400 IU capsules daily; dry form preferred because it is better absorbed.

Selenium: One 100 mcg. tablet or capsule daily.

Colon and Rectal Cancer

Each year, more than one hundred sixty-five thousand people in the United States are diagnosed with colon or rectal cancer, and more than sixty thousand people will die from these diseases. Only 8 percent of all cases of colon and rectal cancer can be attributed to genetics; the rest are due to environmental factors such as diet.

Researchers believe that it is no coincidence that colon and rectal cancer are virtual epidemics in the western world, yet very rare in Asia and Africa. This irrefutable fact strongly suggests that the high-fat, low-fiber diet typical of the west must somehow increase the risk of developing cancer of the colon and rectum.

In fact, several studies have confirmed that people who eat a high-fat diet are at greater risk of developing colon or rectal cancer. For example, in one study of seven thousand men conducted by the Harvard School of Public Health, those who consumed diets that were highest in fat and lowest in fiber were four times more likely to develop *colon polyps,* a precancerous condition. Large epidemiological studies involving thousands of people worldwide confirm that a high-fat, low-fiber diet greatly increases the odds of developing colon or rectal cancer.

In countries where the diet is rich in fiber, people tend to eat many different types of fruits and vegetables throughout the day. Fruits and vegetables are not only packed with fiber, but are filled with other cancer-fighting compounds that may also protect against colon cancer.

Folic acid—For example, folic acid, the B vitamin that has been shown to reduce the risk of cervical cancer, may also protect against colon cancer. In one study, researchers took a dietary survey of 372 people with rectal cancer and 372 cancer-free people. The researchers found that women eating 300 mcg. or more of folic acid daily reduced their risk of colon cancer by more than half, and men eating 385 mcg. of folic acid daily had two-thirds the risk. An interesting sidenote of this study suggests that just one-half cup of spinach per day could supply enough folic acid to reduce the risk of rectal cancer! If you don't eat your spinach, take a folic-acid supplement daily.

Phytic acid—In 1970, British researcher Dr. Denis Burkitt published a study in which he noted that people who live in countries where the fiber intake is high have a astonishingly low rate of colon cancer. Since Dr. Burkitt's observation, many scientists have tried to find the magic bullet in fiber that could provide its anticancer effects. Some speculated that it wasn't one ingredient at all, but the fact that fiber moved food more quickly through the gut, thus reducing exposure to potential carcinogens in food. A growing number of researchers, however, now suspect that fiber may contain a particular ingredient that is a strong anticarcinogen, called *phytic acid*. Phytic acid is an antioxidant compound that is found in many plants, including soy products, cereals, nuts, and legumes. Phytic acid is a *chelator*—that is, it binds with certain metals that may promote tumor growth, thus blocking their negative effect. In laboratory tests, phytic acid was shown to reduce the size and number of tumors in laboratory animals that were fed a potent carcinogen.

Protease Inhibitors—Found in soy foods, protease inhibitors are compounds that block an enzyme that promotes tumor growth. In laboratory experiments, rats were fed a carcinogen known to induce colon cancer and were then fed a protease inhibitor. Test results showed a suppression in the formation of tumors in one hundred percent of the animals, strongly suggesting that protease inhibitors may be a powerful weapon against colon cancer in humans.

Calcium—Calcium, the mineral known for building strong bones, may also reduce the risk of colon cancer. In fact, a nineteen-year study of more than twenty-five thousand people in Chicago found that those who consumed 1200 mg. of calcium daily had a 50 percent reduced risk of colon cancer. Other studies have shown that people who eat a diet rich in calcium produce less amounts of bile acids than people on low-fiber, calcium-poor diets. High levels of bile acids have been associated with a high risk of developing colon cancer.

Earl's Rx

Folic acid: Two 400 mcg. tablets or capsules daily.

Calcium: One 500 mg. calcium with 250 mg. magnesium twice daily, and 400 IU of vitamin D. (In order to maintain the proper balance of minerals, you must take calcium with magnesium. Vitamin D is essential to promote absorption of calcium.)

Soy shake: Protease inhibitors and phytic acid are abundant in soy foods. An easy way to get the full benefit of soy is to drink a soy shake daily. Simply take the right amount of soy powdered beverage (follow directions on label for specific quantity) and blend into 8 ounces of low-fat or no-fat soy milk. Add a few ice cubes and mix in blender. Drink daily as a meal or a between-meals snack.

Personal Advice

I believe that the foods and supplements that I recommend throughout this chapter will help to keep you cancer-free. However, if you have cancer, I feel that it is critical for you to work with an experienced cancer specialist who is also knowledgable in nutrition.

Many forms of cancer today are treatable, especially if they are detected early. Regular check-ups will help to catch any problems early on while the prognosis is still good.

Carpal Tunnel Syndrome

Carpal tunnel syndrome, also called *repetitive stress injury,* accounts for more than half the country's occupational illnesses.

An estimated 185,000 United States office and factory workers a year suffer from some form of this trauma.

Repetitive stress injury costs about 7 billion dollars a year in lost productivity and medical costs.

I f you work on a computer, play a musical instrument, or are in a manual occupation where you perform the same task over and over again, you are at risk of developing Carpal Tunnel Syndrome (CTS). CTS is characterized by pain and numbness in the index and middle fingers, weakness of the thumb, and pain which may be felt in the wrist, palm, and/or forearm. It is caused by the compression of the median nerve as it enters the palm of the hand.

The most common cause of this condition is repetitive overuse of the muscles and tendons of the fingers, hands, arms, and shoulders. Symptoms can be mild such as a sensation of "pins and needles" in the hands, or quite severe such as excruciating pain in the hands, burning and throbbing of the arms, numbness, and weakness. It can sometimes lead to long-term disability.

Typical sufferers are computer programmers, writers and editors, grocery store checkers, factory workers who perform the same repetitive motions every day, and office workers who spend their days in front of a computer keyboard.

Others at increased risk of repetitive stress injuries are menopausal women, pregnant women, women taking oral contraceptives, arthritic patients, diabetics, or kidney patients on hemodialysis. CTS is more prevalent among women and occurs frequently between the ages of forty and sixty years, which leads some experts to suspect that hormonal imbalance may play a role in causing this problem, but the actual role that hormones may play is still unknown.

In severe cases, surgery may be required for CTS, but many cases can be prevented by simple changes in the workplace. In the days before computers put the world at our fingertips, office workers did not have to sit in a chair in front of a screen all day long. They left their posts to distribute mail, work at the photocopy machine, or deliver messages from one employee to another. Today, everything from research to mail to telephone messages to interoffice memos, appear on a screen in front of us, eliminating the need to get up and move around.

As a result, computer users sit in the same position using the same finger movements, sometimes for hours at a time. The same is true in some factory and other labor-intensive jobs where computers and modern technology eliminate unnecessary movement and force workers to sit or stand in the same position all day long.

If you are working in a situation where hand movements are repetitive, here are some work situation guidelines.

Pay attention to the chair. It should slope slightly forward to facilitate proper knee position, keep the back upright or inclined slightly forward from the hips, and should be shaped to maintain the slight natural curve of the lower back. There are several chairs on the market that are specially designed to prevent excess muscle fatigue. Although they cost a bit more than the typical office chair, they are well worth the extra money. Not all chairs are for everybody; be sure to try the chair before you buy it to make sure it is comfortable.

The computer screen should be at or slightly below eye level. The fingers should be able to curve gently and extend from the wrists without having to twist the wrist. The keyboard is best when kept flat for proper wrist positioning and/or just below elbow level. Keep your feet firmly planted on the floor.

Get up every fifteen minutes to stretch or walk around! There is a reason why CTS is called a *repetitive* stress injury. Doing the same task over and over can overuse tired muscles. Simply giving your muscles a break to recover can make a big difference in how you feel at the end of the day.

Studies indicate that a handful of supplements may help to relieve the symptoms of CTS.

Vitamins

Vitamin B6—Some studies have shown that vitamin B6 can be useful in the treatment of CTS, and I have heard many anecdotal reports confirming this. Other studies have shown vitamin B2 to be useful in the treatment of this condition, but the effect is even greater when B6 and B2 are given together.

Herbs

White willow—This natural anti-inflammatory may relieve some of the discomfort in more mild cases of CTS.

Personal Advice

A massage by a well-trained masseuse can help to restore circulation to the shoulders, neck, and arms, which can help to prevent CTS.

Don't underestimate the value of exercise! Anyone who works in a sedentary job, particularly one in which there is repetitive motion, should be involved in a regular strength training program. Exercise not only improves posture, but strength training will strengthen and tone muscles, which can protect against developing CTS.

Earl's Rx

If you are suffering the telltale aches and pains of repetitive stress, try the following.

B-complex with B6: One tablet 50 mg. up to three times daily.

White willow bark: One capsule up to three times daily as needed for pain.

Cataracts

About 4 million people have cataracts, and at least 40,000 people in the United States are blind due to cataracts.

There is compelling new evidence that antioxidants may help to prevent cataracts from forming!

If you've ever tried to look at yourself in a mirror that is clouded with steam, you will have some idea of what it's like to look at the world through eyes that are clouded with cataracts.

A cataract is a clouding of the lens of the eye, which results in the loss of transparency, preventing light from reaching the pupil. A cataract can distort vision by making images appear vague and fuzzy, almost as if you are trying to see through layers of gauze. If the clouding on the eye lens becomes severe, it can result in total blindness of the eye. In many cases, the cataract must be surgically removed. Cataracts exact a steep toll, both on the quality of life of older people and on our pocketbooks. In fact, cataract surgery is so common that it accounts for 12 percent of the Medicare budget!

There are several causes of cataracts, including congenital defects, trauma to the eye, and illnesses such as diabetes. Most cataracts, however, occur as a consequence of aging, specifically due to the exposure over time to free radicals, those overactive oxygen atoms that can destroy healthy tissue.

The eye lens, like many other body tissues, is dependent on adequate levels of antioxidants to prevent damage by free radicals. Studies have shown that cataracts are more common in areas with high annual sunlight levels. Although it is not clear why sunlight exposure may increase the risk of cataracts, scientists believe that when ultraviolet light strikes the eye it naturally causes small particles of oxygen—free radicals—to break off. When these unstable free radicals attach themselves to normal cells in the body (a process called *oxidation*) they injure the cells' membranes. Since eye cells can't regenerate, eye damage caused by oxidation tends to accumulate, eventually causing cataracts.

Recent research has strongly suggested that antioxidants can protect against the cumulative effects of oxidative damage, and may protect against cataracts.

A study conducted at the State University of New York at Stony Brook found that people who consumed plenty of vitamins either by eating fruits and vegetables or by taking multivitamins were 37 percent less likely to have cataracts. The researchers concluded that the antioxidants in fresh produce and/or vitamins have a strong protective effect against cataracts.

Canadian researchers at the University of Western Ontario in London, studied 175 middle-aged people with cataracts and 175 matched controls who did not have the disorder. The researchers reported that the cataract-free individuals had taken at least 400 IU of vitamin E and/or a minimum of 300 mg of vitamin C daily for five years.

Adequate levels of the Vitamin E, selenium, the carotenoids lutein and zeaxanthin, and betacarotene, all of which are found in many fruits and leafy green vegetables, are included in the arsenal of antioxidants necessary to help promote good vision.

Antioxidants

Glutathione—Glutathione is a tripeptide (a combination of three amino acids: glutamate, glycine, and cysteine) that plays an important role in cellular metabolism and protects cells against free-radical injury. It functions as an antioxidant and helps transport vital amino acids to the cells. It is found at very high concentrations in the healthy lens, which led scientists to believe that it is instrumental in protecting the eye. In fact, in animal studies, newborn rats that were given a drug to inhibit the production of glutathione rapidly developed cataracts, which normally does not happen until the animals age.

Vitamin B2 (riboflavin)—Vitamin B2 is essential for the production of glutathione. In one Chinese study, older people who were given a B2 supplement daily had 50 percent fewer cataracts after five years than those who did not take the vitamin.

Vitamin C—Vitamin C also appears to offer significant protection against cataract formation. Studies show that vitamin C levels are high in a normal eye lens, but much lower in a lens with cataracts. In laboratory studies, vitamin C has been found to protect lens proteins and other components of the eye against damage by ultraviolet light. Some researchers believe that in order to fully protect against cataracts, you need to take around 500 mg. of vitamin C daily. To test this hypothesis, the National Eye Institute is sponsoring a long-term study on vitamin C and cataracts, which will be completed in 2001.

Betacarotene—Betacarotene is a member of the carotenoid family, a group of more than 600 compounds found in fruits and vegetables. In a study that followed more than 50,000 nurses over a period of eight years at Brigham and Women's Hospital in Boston, researchers found that women whose diets were rich in betacarotene were 40 percent less likely to develop cataracts than those whose diets were low in this important vitamin.

Lutein—Lutein is also a member of the carotenoid family and is found in great concentration in the *macula* of the eye, the back part of the retina where entering light hits and send signals to the brain. Lutein is also a potent antioxidant, which leads some researchers to hypothesize that it is concentrated in the eye for a reason, that is, to protect it from oxidative damage.

Vitamin E—According to a Finnish study published in the *British Medical Journal,* people with low blood levels of vitamin E are nearly twice as likely to develop cataracts as people with normal levels.

Herbs

Bilberry—Used by herbalist for years to treat various eye problems, this herb may help to prevent cataracts. In one study, bilberry extract plus vitamin E stopped the progression of cataract formation in 97 percent of fifty older patients with cataracts. Bilberry was also used by British fighter pilots during World War II who claimed that it helped relieve night blindness!

Personal Advice

I never go out in the bright sun without a good pair of sunglasses, and neither should you. Avoid exposure of the eyes to high-energy radiation (direct sunlight) by wearing sunglasses (make sure that they block both UVB and UVA light) and a hat with a brim during peak sunlight hours.

Avoid smoking; it promotes the formation of free radicals. Consume free-radical scavengers such as vitamins E, C and betacarotene, and consume antioxidants that help absorb UV light such as betacarotene, lutein, and zeaxanthin.

Fruits and vegetables are a good source of antioxidants, especially the dark green vegetables such as spinach, peppers, and broccoli. Vegetables rich in vitamin A include squash and sweet potatoes. Carrots and winter squash are excellent sources of betacarotene. One raw carrot contains 13,500 IU of betacarotene—more than 250 percent of the RDA. Winter squash is not only rich in betacarotene, it has an extra bonus: It's rich in potassium and it is chock full of vitamin C.

Keeping diabetes under control is critical. Diabetes can increase the risk of developing cataracts by more than 400 percent in people under the age of 65. (See "Diabetes," page 111.)

Earl's Rx

Combination cataract-buster multivitamin supplement: There are many specially designed supplements for eye health on the market today that combine the necessary antioxidants. These formulas typically include B2, selenium, alpha and betacarotene, lutein, vitamins C and E, B-complex, and zinc. The usual dose is one or two tablets or capsules daily, as directed.

In addition to the multivitamin supplement, I also recommend the following.

Glutathione: Two 500 mg. capsules daily on an empty stomach.

Bilberry: One capsule up to three times daily.

Chronic Fatigue Syndrome

Chronic fatigue syndrome (CFS) may affect as many as 5 million people in the U.S.

Sufferers are predominately young adult women, but the condition occurs in people of all ages, races, and sexes.

There is no proven treatment, but improving general health through diet, adequate rest, and exercise is helpful.

You feel tired even after you've had enough sleep. You drag yourself through the morning, push yourself to get through the rest of the day, then fall asleep exhausted before the nightly news is over. You go to the doctor who does a quick examination and then recommends more rest or tells you to take a vacation. You know that isn't going to help. You feel helpless, resentful that the doctor hasn't taken you more seriously, and wonder if it's all in your mind.

Most likely, your doctor is just as frustrated as you are because fatigue is one of the most common complaints doctors hear. There is probably no other symptom that has more possible causes than fatigue. It can be the most apparent indication of depression, cancer, insomnia, anemia, low blood pressure, viral infection, Lupus, Lyme disease, multiple sclerosis, arthritis, inner-ear imbalance, hypoglycemia, hypertension, cardiac disease—the list is endless.

But Chronic Fatigue Syndrome (CFS) is much more than merely feeling tired; it is a particular problem characterized by unexplained debilitating fatigue which lasts for more than six months, and is not due to any other underlying physical problem. Patients with CFS often have a combination of symptoms, including sore throat, swollen glands, low-grade fever, muscle pain, and sometimes confusion. These symptoms may come and go, resulting in even more difficulty in diagnosing the condition. Since fatigue is such a general symptom, anyone who suffers from excessive fatigue should be seen by a doctor for a thorough workup.

In fact, it wasn't until 1988 that the Centers for Disease Control and Prevention officially described the syndrome. Even today, some doctors don't believe the syndrome exists and that those who complain of its symptoms may actually either be faking or suffering from depression.

A study reported in *Annals of Medicine* (1994) looked into possible causes of CFS. One theory is that chronic fatigue syndrome is a lasting specific immune dysfunction that was originally induced by a viral infection. Epstein-Barr virus, herpes simplex virus, and Coxsackie B virus, are among the viruses that have been suspected, but have not been proven to cause fatigue.

Unfortunately, there is no one diagnostic test for this problem, therefore, it must be diagnosed based on specific criteria. In order to receive a diagnosis of chronic fatigue syndrome, you must have experienced the following:

- Sudden onset of persistent, unexplained chronic tiredness (it cannot be a lifelong problem).

- Fatigue that is not relieved by rest.

- Difficulty concentrating and remembering facts severely enough to impair your ability to work.

- Tenderness in the lymph nodes in the neck and/or under the arms.

- Muscle pain and pain in the joints without swelling or redness.

- Headaches of a new type, pattern, or severity.

- Unrefreshing sleep.

Some studies have linked extreme stress, such as a death in the family or divorce, as factors that may contribute to the onset of chronic fatigue syndrome. Although there is no concrete evidence that this is true, we do know that stress can have a profound effect on the immune system, our body's natural defense against disease. If the immune system is weakened, it could leave the body vulnerable to infection.

A groundbreaking study that was published in the *Journal of the American Medical Association* appears to be a major breakthrough in revealing the cause of chronic fatigue syndrome in many patients. The study, which included twenty-three patients with chronic fatigue syndrome, found that twenty-two of them had an abnormality in the way their bodies regulated blood pressure, which caused their hearts to slow down at precisely the times when it needed to speed up. For example, during periods of exertion, for instance, when you get up from a chair, you need a stronger heartbeat to pump blood throughout the body. In the patients with chronic fatigue syndrome, however, the heartbeat did not speed up when it should have and actually slowed down. Oddly enough, this particular kind of low blood pressure cannot be diagnosed by the standard blood-pressure test. Instead, the patient must be tilted at a 70-degree angle to the floor to simulate standing for a long period of time, the kind of exertion which can trigger the low blood-pressure response. According to this study, during the tilt test, the patients with chronic fatigue syndrome and low blood pressure experienced light-headedness, faintness and nausea, and may have felt lethargic and fatigued for days after the test. Researchers believe that if this low blood-pressure response occurs often enough during the day, it might be the cause of the continual exhaustion.

Most of the patients in the study were successfully treated with medication and an increased intake of salt and fluid to control blood pressure. Out of the twenty-two patients who had low blood pressure, nine reported full recovery after treatment and seven said that their condition had improved.

Not every patient with this type of low blood pressure develops chronic fatigue syndrome. This has led researchers to speculate that a viral infection or some other illness must somehow trigger chronic fatigue syndrome in people with this kind of low blood pressure, and perhaps this condition makes people susceptible to chronic fatigue syndrome. The CFS story is far from over: More studies are needed to determine if low blood pressure is truly the cause of chronic fatigue syndrome in many patients.

In the meantime, there are few effective treatments for chronic fatigue syndrome. Supplements that help control inflammation may help to relieve the headache and muscle pain. Antidepressants have also been helpful for many patients, and many others have found relief by practicing relaxation techniques, such as yoga and deep breathing. Keep in mind that with CFS the symptoms tend not to worsen over time, and there is no evidence of long-term physical deterioration. In fact, many people with this problem eventually recover.

Here are some supplements that may help fight fatigue and increase energy levels.

Amino Acids

L-carnitine—Could a deficiency in L-carnitine be a factor in CFS? A recent study reported in *Clinical Infectious Diseases* (1994), evaluated thirty-eight patients with chronic fatigue syndrome and 308 healthy patients for L-carnitine levels. Generally, those with chronic fatigue have lower blood levels of L-carnitine, and those who recovered from the syndrome subsequently raised their levels of carnitine. L-carnitine is derived from the essential amino acids, L-lysine and methionine, and is important in energy production. The researchers concluded that an evaluation of carnitine levels can be an important tool in diagnosing chronic fatigue syndrome. I have long recommended L-carnitine for sufferers of fatigue of any kind, and feel that it may be particularly helpful in CFS.

Enzymes

Coenzyme Q10—Coenzyme Q10 is important for the production of energy by all cells in the body. Athletes take CoQ10 supplements for increased endurance. Good food sources are mackerel, bran, sesame, legumes, sardines, spinach, and peanuts. Foods lose CoQ10 through processing, storage, and cooking; fresh foods are best. CoQ10 is also available in supplement form.

Herbs

Siberian ginseng—Ginseng has been used by Asian healers for more than five thousand years as a tonic herb for overall health, and as a stimulant and energy booster. The Chinese use it to treat dozens of ailments including the treatment of fatigue and exhaustion. There are several types of ginseng—I personally recommend Siberian ginseng, which is a botanical cousin to Asian ginseng and has many of the same properties without any of the negative side effects. (Some people find that Asian ginseng can make them too hyper and can cause insomnia.)

In the late 1950s and 1960s, Eastern European researchers documented ginseng's mental and physical antifatigue effects in both animal trials and double-blind clinical trials in humans. Some researchers attribute CFS to a general immune-system failure, and Siberian ginseng is reputed to normalize impaired immune functions. In fact, studies note that Siberian ginseng appears to activate the immune system, and may increase the number and effectiveness of disease fighting cells, helper T-cells and natural killer cells. Both of these effects could be put to good use in the treatment of chronic fatigue syndrome.

Suma—This South American version of ginseng was first used by Brazilian Indian tribes. In South America it is used as a tonic. In North America, it has been used to treat exhaustion resulting from debilitating viral infections.

DHEA—Short for dehydroepiandrosterone, DHEA is now available over the counter and is reputed to be a potent energy tonic. I have heard several anecdotal reports of DHEA helping to relieve the fatigue and lethargy typical of CFS.

Personal advice

It's not surprising that victims of CFS are primarily female. Today's "superwoman" who balances career, home, family, and social life suffers from an acute shortage of time. The result is a constant state of stress and sleep deprivation. Get off the treadmill for a few days and evaluate your lifestyle. Look seriously at how you can reduce your workload. Make sure you are getting enough sleep, prioritize your schedule, set limits, pace yourself.

Low blood sugar (*hypoglycemia*) is another culprit that can cause fatigue. Cut out too many sugars and other refined carbohydrates, and increase your intake of protein. Coffee is a stimulant that can fool you into thinking it gives you energy, but once you break the caffeine addiction, you are likely to feel more energetic.

When evaluation by a physician cannot find a physical cause for exhaustion, look to your diet. Are you eating enough of the right foods to maintain your energy throughout the day? Just as a car needs fuel to run, the body needs fuel to keep going.

We get energy from food in the form of calories. In today's society, where there is a great emphasis on weight and body fat, *calorie* has become a dirty word. Some people misunderstand and simply do not take in enough calories to give the body what it needs to keep all its organs in proper chemical balance.

Most adults need between 1300 and 1400 calories a day just to stay alive without any physical activity. How many additional calories you need depends on what you do all day—the more activity, the more calories.

The trick is to eat foods that promote good health. Calories from grains, poultry, fish, eggs, beans, nuts, soy products, vegetables, and fruit are certainly preferable to those from fat, sugar, refined flours, and most snack foods.

Exercise will increase your caloric needs, but it is a great energy booster and stress reliever. Make some form of nonstressful exercise part of your daily routine.

Earl's Rx

Boost your energy with these supplements.

L-carnitine: One 500 mg. capsule, twice daily between meals.

Coenzyme Q10: 30–100 mg. daily, available in capsules.

Siberian ginseng: 500 mg. capsule, up to three times daily. Take one half-hour before or after meals.

Suma: One 500 mg. capsule, up to three times daily.

DHEA: One 25 mg. tablet or capsule daily.

Colds

Colds are the single most common ailment affecting humans.

The common cold may be caused by nearly one hundred different viruses.

Preschool children are the most susceptible, contracting as many as six colds a year. The average adult has two or three colds a year.

The common cold: It's not serious or life-threatening, but it can certainly make your life miserable. The common cold is a viral infection of the upper-respiratory tract that attacks the nose and nasal passages, and can spread to the chest.

We all know and dread those first symptoms: the scratchy throat, sneezing, headache, aching muscles, and congestion. There is no magic potion that can spare us the misery of the next four to ten days of runny noses, coughing, sleeplessness—and in severe cases, bronchitis or sinus infection. There are however, several natural treatments that may help relieve symptoms and shorten the duration of the cold.

Vitamins

Vitamin C—My friend and colleague, the late Linus Pauling, may have won the Nobel Prize for his work in physics, but the renowned scientist also knew his vitamin C. Dr. Pauling was the first to sing the praises of vitamin C as a treatment for the common cold and, indeed, decades later, he has been proven right. In twenty-one separate studies, vitamin C reduced the length and severity of symptoms of the common cold by an average of 23 percent.

Vitamin C's benefit in fighting the common cold may be due to its antioxidant properties. When an infection strikes, special cells in the immune system release large amounts of oxidizing materials that can be toxic to other cells. Activation of these cells promotes the consumption of vitamin C in the body, suggesting that high concentrations of the vitamin may provide protection against the harmful effects of the toxins that are released.

Vitamin A—Vitamin A lowers the risk of severe respiratory infections. After analyzing twenty controlled studies, researchers reported in the *British Medical Journal* (1993) that vitamin A supplements reduced deaths from respiratory disease by 70 percent. For a bad cold or respiratory infection, increase your intake of betacarotene, which is converted to vitamin A as the body needs it. (High dosages of pure vitamin A can be toxic and are not recommended.)

Minerals

Zinc—Zinc is well-known for wound healing and as a stimulant to the body's immune system, but a recent study that tested zinc against the common cold indicates that although zinc does not kill the nasty viruses responsible for the cold, it seems to prevent the virus from reproducing or duplicating itself.

In one study, over seventy Dartmouth students sucked on flavored zinc-glyconate-glycine lozenges within one day of the first sign of a cold. Those who took the lozenges every two hours four times a day got rid of their colds more quickly than those who did not.

Herbs

Echinacea—Echinacea, the Native-American herb derived from the roots of *Echinacea angustifolia* or the roots or leaves of echinacea, is an increasingly popular herb that has received much attention lately. If taken when symptoms first appear, echinacea works as an anti-inflammatory and antiinfectious agent that can help to relieve symptoms.

A clinical study of 180 male and female patients between the ages of eighteen and sixty found that four droppersful of a standard extract of echinacea root (the kind that is sold in natural-food stores) had a significant effect in relieving symptoms and duration of colds and flulike infections.

Elderberry—This herb has recently been shown to be an immune enhancer that can help to ward off colds.

Elm bark—This soother of irritating coughs and *demulcent* (loosens mucous) should be given as a tea or in lozenges.

Rose hips—These fruits are a good source of vitamin C, and can be given as a tea or a supplement.

Goldenseal—This herb has antibacterial properties, and was used by Native Americans to treat infections. It can be taken internally or used as a gargle.

Camphor, menthol, and euclyptol—These plant derivatives are excellent for nasal congestion.

Siberian ginseng—A botanical cousin of the illustrious ginseng family, it has many medicinal qualities. Siberian ginseng has been used to treat bronchitis and chronic lung ailments and helps cure colds and infections.

Anise—This spice has also been used a remedy since the time of the ancient Egyptians. Among its many uses, it helps loosen phlegm and to fight coughs and colds.

Bayberry bark—It has been used for decades for a variety of ills. A hot tea made from the powdered bark of the bayberry taken at the first sign of a cold, cough, or flu, is an excellent expectorant. It also promotes perspiration, which allows you to literally sweat out a cold.

Nettle—Nettle is a well-known folk remedy for hay fever and other allergies. It helps relieve inflammation caused by allergic reactions and clears congestion in the nose and chest. (Do not use nettle if you are pregnant or have kidney disease without first checking with your physician.)

Cayenne (also known as capsicum)—This substance found in peppers contains more vitamin C than oranges. Cayenne tea is excellent for colds and chills.

Ephedra—Medicinal use of this herb dates back to about 2800 B.C. when Chinese healers used it in the treatment of the common cold, asthma, hay fever, bronchitis, and other ailments. Western medicine's use of the herb began in 1923 when a compound found in ephedra, *ephedrine*, was demonstrated to possess a number of pharmacological effects and was soon synthesized. Since then, ephedrine has been used since for symptomatic relief for asthma, hay fever, and runny nose. **(If you use ephedra products, you should do so under the supervision of your**

physician or natural healer. If taken in high enough doses, ephedra can cause fatal heart problems.)

Peppermint—Peppermint has been used for medicinal purposes for thousands of years by ancient Egyptians, Greeks, and Romans, primarily for the treatment of indigestion and intestinal colic as well as in the treatment of colds, fever, and headache.

Personal Advice

We all want to be mothered when we have a cold; maybe that's because those comforting home remedies that were passed on from generation to generation work! Here are a few examples.

Nose drops made with 1/4 teaspoon of salt with four ounces of warm water will help unstuff your child's nose.

A humidifier adds soothing moisture to a room, but be sure it's clean and mold-free. Add aromatic herbs (sage, eucalyptus, thyme, rosemary, or wintergreen) to a pot of boiling water, let steep for about fifteen minutes, and then inhale the steam for relief of congestion.

In addition, the oil of eucalyptus and its active ingredient, *eucalyptol,* are frequently found in over-the-counter cough drops and salves.

Reach for the chicken soup—Researchers have proven that grandma was right! Drinking chicken soup is more effective than drinking hot water or other liquids for the relief nasal congestion. *The New England Journal of Medicine* confirmed what every mother already knows—chicken soup is a mild antibiotic and decongestant and is effective against the common cold. Chinese healers also use chicken soup to treat colds, but they add a little ginseng. And don't forget Grandma also knew about the abilities of onion and garlic to alleviate congestion and help a persistent cough. Add some onion and garlic cloves to your chicken stock.

If you find you are catching a lot of colds, remember, a healthy body is the first defense against disease. Get enough sleep. Studies have shown that even missing one night's sleep can depress your immune system. Exercise and eat well—look for foods that contain the antioxidants the body needs. These include dark-green leafy vegetables, yellow and orange vegetables, fruit, liver, milk, nuts, seeds, whole grains, wheat germ, citrus fruits, tomatoes, broccoli, green peppers, strawberries, melons, cabbage, beans, eggs, and enriched breads and cereals.

Don't wait until the symptoms are completely debilitating—start treatment at the first sign of a cold. Get extra rest and, if possible, cut back on your usual schedule for a few days to give your body a chance to heal.

Earl's Rx

Here's what I do when I feel a cold coming on.

Vitamin C: Four 500 mg. capsules of calcium ascorbate daily. For best results, take two with breakfast and two later in the day with food.

Betacarotene: Take one 25,000–50,000 IU capsule or tablet daily for three to four days.

Echincea: Take one to three doses of 500 mg. daily.

Garlic: Take one to three odorless garlic capsules for three to four days.

Elderberry: Take one or two 500 mg. elderberry capsules or liquid daily until symptoms abate.

Cystitis

Cystitis is primarily a woman's disease, but it can also affect men

Twenty percent of all women will suffer from an episode of cystitis at some time during their lifetimes.

C ystitis (also known as *bladder infection*) is the inflammation of the urinary tract, most often caused by infection. The most common culprit is *E. coli*, the intestinal bacteria that is vital to maintaining intestinal health, but devastating when the bacteria enters the urethra and makes its way to the bladder.

The reason women are twenty-five times more vulnerable to bladder infections than are men is due to simple anatomical differences. Because the female bladder is much shorter than the male urethra, E. coli have an easy time reaching the female bladder. When you don't drink enough fluids to wash them away, the microorganisms adhere to the bladder walls and begin multiplying. The results? An intense urge to urinate, burning during urination and, in some cases, blood in the urine, which can be very frightening.

Allopathic medicine uses antibiotics as the first line of defense, specifically the drugs Bactrim, Septra, or Cipro. Antibiotics will help prevent a simple bladder infection from turning into a life-threatening kidney infection, and are often necessary once the infection takes hold. The problem with antibiotics, however, is that they are not selective and kill as many good bacteria as bad bacteria. This, in turn, alters the body's normal balance of microorganisms and because the microorganisms are altered, the conditions are also optimal for vaginal yeast infections. To make matters worse, for many women cystitis is a chronic condition, so they must take antibiotics frequently. To add to their misery, these women run the risk of developing antibiotic-resistant infections, as well as yeast infections.

If you have a tendency to contract cystitis, a combination of common sense and supplements may help to prevent a recurrence.

Herbs

Cranberry—For years, women have sworn by cranberry juice as means of alleviating the frequency and duration of cystitis and for years, researchers were puzzled as to why it worked. Now, medical researchers have confirmed that the cranberry is much more than a fruit to eat on Thanksgiving; it is also a potent infection fighter. A group of Boston-based scientists looked at two groups of elderly women who often show urine that contains bacteria and white-blood cells—signs that an infection may be in the making. One group drank 10 ounces of cranberry juice a day while the other consumed the same amount of a placebo beverage that looked and tasted the same, but contained no cranberry juice.

After about six weeks, a percentage of those who drank the cranberry juice showed a drop in bacteria and white-blood cells in their urine; the count remained low during the entire six-month study. Those who had the placebo showed no change. While all researchers do not agree on why cranberry juice fights cystitis, one current theory is that a substance in cranberry juice keeps the problem bacteria from clinging to the wall of the urinary tract, thus literally flushing it out in the urine. Cranberry also contains compounds called *anthocyanosides,* which are natural antibiotics; these may also help to keep these troublesome bacteria under control. (Anthocyanosides are also present in blueberries.)

Since pure cranberry juice might be too tart for some, most manufacturers also sell a blend of juice, water, and sugar. Look for the low-sugar blend if you need to drink a lot of cranberry juice; sugar nourishes the offending bacteria. The easiest and simplest way to get the full benefit of cranberry without the added sugar is by taking capsules.

Garlic—The herb that stops vampires in their tracks is also lethal to bacteria and viruses. Garlic contains a compound called *allicin,* which not only kills bacteria but is especially effective against microorganisms that can cause yeast infections.

Acidophilus—If you are on antibiotics, you run the risk of getting a yeast infection. (See "Vaginal Yeast Infections," page 262.) Acidophilus culture helps the body to maintain a normal balance between good and bad bacteria, which not only keeps infection at bay but also helps to get rid of yeast infections. If you are taking antibiotics for any reason, eat yogurt or take acidophilus supplements for a couple of weeks to reestablish healthy bowel flora.

Uva ursi—More than a thousand years ago, the Chinese and Native Americans were using uva ursi to treat urinary tract infections in both men and women. This herb contains a substance called *arbutin*, which is converted in the urine to *hydroquinone*, a urinary antiseptic. Uva ursi is a natural diuretic—it literally flushes out the kidneys. If you use uva ursi regularly, you will need to replenish potassium, which can be lost when you lose fluid. Be sure to eat foods high in potassium, or take a potassium supplement.

Cinnamon—This spice not only adds flavor to cookies, puddings, and apple cider, but is also a natural antiseptic. Sprinkle liberally on fruit and cereal.

Alfalfa—First discovered by the Arabs, who dubbed this valuable plant the "father of all foods," the leaves of the alfalfa plant are rich in minerals and nutrients. What makes this herb particularly good for cystitis is that it is an excellent diuretic, promoting urination and thus helping to rid the body of bad bacteria.

Barberry—This fruit contains a compound called *berberine*, a natural antibiotic. Recent studies have confirmed the infection-fighting properties of berberine; it is effective against E coli which causes urinary tract infections. (Berberine is also found in goldenseal, another natural antibiotic.)

Personal Advice

Get enough fluid—As part of any healthy diet, drink six to eight glasses of water a day and minimize your intake of alcohol and caffeine. Don't make a habit of holding in your urine. Urinate every two to three hours.

Diet tips—Cut back on your intake of refined starches and sugars, vegetable fats, onions, beans, and chocolate.

Sexual practices—Urinate before and after having sex (keeping the bladder full during intercourse can be very irritating). Some women have frequent attacks of cystitis after intercourse. In some cases, these flareups might be due to the use of a diaphragm, which can press against the urethra if it is not properly fitted. Other women may find latex condoms irritating. If you suffer from frequent attacks of cystitis, talk to your physician about the best method of contraception for you.

It is not advisable to have sex when you are in the midst of a cystitis flare-up; it may further aggravate your problem, and there is a risk that you may pass the problem onto your partner.

Avoid irritants—Do not use oils, feminine hygiene sprays, or talcum powder in your genital area, and don't douche with any chemical substances. Avoid bath oils or bubble baths; take showers instead.

During menstruation, change sanitary napkins and tampons frequently. Both have been known to provide a route for bacteria. In addition, tampons may put pressure on the urethra, encouraging infection.

Wear cotton underpants—avoid synthetic fibers that can block the proper circulation of air and promote the growth of bacteria. Change into dry clothes as soon as possible after swimming, and be sure to thoroughly dry the genital area after bathing. Keep in mind that bacteria need a warm, moist area to flourish, and you want to make your body as inhospitable as possible!

Earl's Rx

Cranberry: Drink one glass of unsweetened juice daily or take cranberry capsules (400 mg.) three times daily.

Garlic: Two raw, aged odorless garlic capsules daily.

Uva ursi: One to three 500 mg. capsules daily.

Barberry: One to three capsules daily.

Depression

Depression is the most common of all emotional disorders.

Extreme stress can trigger depression. Recent research shows that some people are biologically programmed to react with depression when they are overstressed.

Poor diet and nutritional deficiencies can contribute to feeling blue.

Nearly all of us have felt depressed at some point in our lives and, very often, within a short time we bounce back to normal. But when the depression doesn't lift within a week or two, it may a sign of *clinical depression*, a bona fide health problem that may worsen if it is not effectively treated. Symptoms are wide-ranging and are often mistaken for other ailments. Common signs of depression include insomnia, digestive problems, fatigue, headache, muscle pain, forgetfulness, lack of ability to concentrate, weight loss or gain, and withdrawal from social and business life.

In fact, so many ailments can be traced to depression that it is often difficult to sort out the physical from the emotional; it is generally accepted that physical wellbeing cannot be separated from our feelings and emotions. This link between the two is not difficult to understand; science has shown that extreme stress can actually weaken the ability of the immune system to fight disease, just as a severe illness can trigger a major depression. In my experience, I have also seen cases in which nutritional deficiencies have contributed to depression, and when the right combination of diet and supplements has made a real and palpable difference.

Why do so many of us get depressed? Depression may be caused by a wide range of factors, including childhood traumas or current events, such as the loss of a job or a loved one. But almost all depression is characterized by feelings of helplessness and loss of control over your life.

Recently, researchers have been investigating the physical causes of depression, that is, whether certain chemical changes may contribute or trigger depression. In fact, there is some evidence that deficiency in certain key chemical nerve transmitters in the brain, such as the catecholamines and serotonin, accompanies depression. What is unclear is which comes first—the depression or the biological changes.

Anyone who is feeling depressed for more than a week or two should seek help from a physician or natural healer. Denying the symptoms won't make them go away, and the right kind of help at the right time can make a huge difference in how you feel.

Although depression can be triggered by many different factors, a recent study links low blood pressure to a tendency to become depressed. According to an intriguing study reported in the *British Medical Journal* (1994) having low blood pressure may contribute to or, in fact, actually cause depression. In a study of 846 men sixty to eighty years of age, those with low blood pressure showed increased signs of depression, including feelings of sadness, fatigue, and loss of appetite. Interestingly, a recent study also linked low blood pressure to chronic fatigue syndrome, a physical problem that also is characterized by depression. In this case, the solution was fairly simple: Raising the low blood pressure to more normal levels helped reduce the symptoms of chronic fatigue. If you have low blood pressure and are feeling depressed, you should see your physician or natural healer for possible treatment.

How is depression treated? A combination of psychotherapy (the talking cure) and medication is usually helpful in treating depression. In recent years, there has been great emphasis on curing the problem by prescribing one of three different types of antidepressant medications. They include *serotonin reuptake inhibitors,* which are drugs that affect several of the brain's chemical messengers; *tricylic antidepressants,* which are thought to work by increasing the availability of another brain chemical called *norepinephine;* and *MAO inhibitors,* which prevent the activity of the enzyme monoamine oxidase in brain tissue and therefore affect moods. As a pharmacist, I know that for people who are suffering from acute depression these drugs can be true lifesavers. But there are also some significant downsides to these drugs. I have heard people complain bitterly about the potential side effects, including some downright unpleasant ones such as dry mouth, abnormal heart rate, difficulty in urinating, bloating, confusion, difficulty in achieving erection, and loss of libido in both sexes. In addition, the long-term effects of these drugs are unknown. That is why I recommend trying simple things first. In cases of mild depression, some natural remedies may offer relief with few if any side effects. Here are some to consider.

Herbs

St. John's wort—For years, I have been telling people that this herb is an excellent antidepressant, and about how it has been used in Europe quite successfully to treat cases of mild depression. Recently, I was gratified to see that the prestigious *British Medical Journal* agreed. In an article that reviewed more than thirty separate studies, researchers concluded that St. John's wort was as effective an antidepressant as many stronger prescription medications. This herb has been the subject of several studies, most of them performed in Europe. In one study, 105 depressed patients, twenty to sixty-four years old, were treated for four weeks with either an extract of St. John's wort or a placebo. By the end of the study, more than two-thirds of the St. John's wort group showed improvement, versus only 28 percent in the placebo group. The researchers concluded that St. John's wort had an antidepressive effect in the treatment of mild and moderate depression that was at least as effective as some traditional antidepressants, but without any undesirable side effects.

Kava kava—This member of the pepper family is found mainly in Micronesia, Melanesia, and Polynesia. Several European countries have approved kava preparations in the treatment of nervous anxiety, insomnia, and restlessness. I know from personal experience that this herb can restore peace of mind and tranquility, and can promote a feeling of wellbeing.

Ginkgo biloba—This well-researched herb improves the circulation to the brain and can be an effective mood elevator.

Siberian ginseng—These are at least five different plants that go by the name ginseng and, although all are tonics, they all have different properties. Studies in Russia indicate that *Siberian ginseng* (a botanical cousin of Asian ginseng), along with being an energy tonic, has a positive effect on stress and depression. Unlike other forms of ginseng, which may give some people too much of a lift, Siberian ginseng does not promote insomnia.

Vitamins

B-complex—B vitamins are nature's antidote to stress, and since stress can lead to depression, it is important to keep yourself fortified by getting enough B. Many of the symptoms of depression that are found in the elderly, such as confusion, memory loss, and apathy, are actually due to a deficiency in vitamin B12. In fact, as many as 10 percent of all people over sixty may have low blood levels of this vitamin. Due to changes in digestion, people over 60 may not be able to absorb B12 from their food, so a supplement is essential.

Other supplements

DHEA—This hormone, which is produced in the adrenal glands, brain, and skin, is a natural mood enhancer that may help to prevent mild depression. As we age, our levels of DHEA decline. In one study recently conducted at the University of San Diego, for three months thirteen men and seventeen women aged forty to seventy took a DHEA supplement sufficient to restore their blood levels to those of young adults. For another three months, the participants received a placebo. Neither the researchers nor the subjects knew who was taking DHEA or the placebo at any given time. The researchers found that when the participants were taking DHEA, they reported a "remarkable increase in perceived physical and psychological wellbeing for both men and women." In other words, when they were on DHEA, the participants felt better, a lot better. In particular, people on DHEA say that they experienced increased energy, better sleep, felt more relaxed, and were better able to handle stress.

Omega-3 fatty acids—We know that lowering high cholesterol is good for your physical health, but what about your mental health? Several years ago, in a highly publicized study, researchers linked a reduction in blood cholesterol with increased depression leading to suicide. Further confusion resulted when subsequent studies showed just the opposite, that is, in these later studies, people who follow cholesterol-lowering diets end up *less* depressed than they were initially. Why did researchers reach such different conclusions?

According to an article published in the *American Journal of Clinical Nutrition,* the answer may lie in the type of food that is eaten on a low-fat diet and, more specifically, whether the low-fat diet includes ample amounts of a long chain polyunsaturated fatty acids like docosahexaenoic acid or DHA, an omega-3 fatty acid, which is found in cold-water fish. The study's author, Dr. Joseph Hibbeln, a psychiatrist with the National Institute of Alcohol Abuse and Alcoholism, noted that in one study of people living in the coastal areas of Finland where fish is a mainstay, there was no evidence of depression when these people went on a low-fat diet. However, in other studies involving inland residents, there was a marked increase in depression among people on low-fat diets, which typically did not include much fish.

Why do certain types of fish protect against depression? Studies strongly suggest that DHA, the fatty acid found in fish, is essential for normal mental function. These fatty acids may have many jobs in the body, including a possible role in the production of neurotransmitters. In fact, research has shown that primates fed a diet low in this particular fat actually became more violent and aggressive. The same may be true for humans. To bolster his theory, Dr. Hibbeln cites statistics that show that the rates of depression have risen steadily over the decades as the proportion of this particular type of fatty acid in the diet has declined. A case in point: The most popular forms of fat in the United States, margarine and processed vegetable oils, are high in omega-6 fatty acids, and low in omega-3.

The solution to the low-fat–depression spiral is an easy one: eat more fatty fish (salmon, halibut, sea bass, albacore tuna, and sardines) or take a fish oil supplement!

Personal Advice

Burn away those blues—Exercise can have important psychological benefits for those suffering from depression. Exercise triggers the release of *endophins,* nature's own painkillers, which produces a feeling of well-being. Two studies demonstrated that aerobic exercise plus counseling was more effective in the treatment of depressive disorders than counseling alone.

Most important, don't ignore symptoms of depression. Find the therapy that will work for you. Exercise is a great stress reducer and should be included in your daily regimen. Look for those supplements that help you relax, regulate sleep patterns, and promote a sense of well-being.

Earl's Rx

If you are prone to mild depression, these supplements should help to give you a much needed boost.

The basic Bs: One 50 mg. B-complex capsule or tablet, one 500 mg. B1 (thiamine) capsule or tablet, and one 1000 mcg. B12 (sublingual form) daily.

St. John's wort: One capsule, three times daily.

Kava kava: One capsule, three times daily.

Gingko biloba: One 60 mg. capsule or tablet, up to three times daily.

Siberian ginseng: One or two 500 mg. capsules daily.

Omega-3 fatty acids: One 1000 mg. capsule up to six times daily.

DHEA: One 25 mg. tablet or capsule daily.

Diabetes

14 million Americans are diabetic.

The older you are, the greater the risk you have of developing diabetes.

If you live in the United States, you are much more likely to develop diabetes than if you lived in any of the Mediterranean countries, South America, or Asia. Why? Diet and lifestyle are critical factors. Americans eat too much of the wrong food, too little of the right food, and consume far too few of the supplements that can help to keep diabetes under control.

Diabetes is a general term that refers to a group of biochemical disorders characterized by the body's inability to utilize the carbohydrates, sugars, and starches that are found in food. As a result, blood-sugar levels rise, which can lead to other serious problems including heart disease, stroke, kidney disease, and blindness. Early warning signs include excessive production of urine, constant thirst, and weight loss.

Two types of diabetes are the most common: They are type I (also known as *juvenile onset diabetes*) and type II (also known as *adult onset diabetes.*) As its name implies, juvenile diabetes strikes during childhood and is caused by the failure of the pancreas to produce enough insulin, the hormone that breaks down glucose or sugar so that it can be utilized by body cells. Type I diabetes is typically treated with supplemental insulin, as well as a carefully restricted, low-sugar diet. If you are born with type I diabetes or develop it early in life, you will require medical attention by a qualified physician, preferably one who specializes in diabetes.

Type II diabetes is an entirely different problem: It is a problem of *insulin resistance*. In other words, the body produces enough insulin, but the insulin does not work efficiently. Although it is usually not considered as serious as type I diabetes, type II diabetes can lead to many serious health problems, including kidney disease, nerve damage, and blindness, and should be treated aggressively.

Clearly, a diagnosis of type II diabetes should not be taken lightly, but as a sign that it is time to make some constructive changes in your life. Fortunately, there are many things that you can do to thwart the progression of this disease and, perhaps, to prevent it from occurring in the first place.

Obesity (being 20 percent or more overweight) is a major risk factor for type II diabetes. In fact, 95 percent of diabetics are overweight. The right diet can go a long way in helping to control diabetes and to prevent obesity, a major risk factor for this disease.

For example, adding more fish to your diet may help to prevent the onset of diabetes. A Dutch study followed 175 people between the ages of sixty-four and eighty-seven for three years, and found that the fish eaters were least likely to develop glucose intolerance, an early sign of insulin resistance and a precursor of diabetes. As little as an ounce of fish per day was linked to this benefit.

Trimming the fat will also definitely help to ward of diabetes, as well as heart disease. When researchers tracked 123 people with glucose intolerance for up to three years, they found that those who ate the most fat were the most likely to develop diabetes. Researchers noted that an extra 40 grams of fat a day increased the risk of developing diabetes by *six times* in people with elevated blood sugar. As reported in *Diabetes Care* (January, 1994), people who developed diabetes consumed 43 percent of the day's calories from fat, while people who kept diabetes at bay consumed about 38 percent of calories from fat. From this study we can see that even a small amount of extra fat can have serious consequences on our health. (Keep in mind that a diet of 38 percent fat is still too high; I recommend consuming no more than 20 percent of your daily calories in the form of fat.)

Whether you have type I or type II diabetes, following a careful diet can prevent your condition from worsening. In addition to a careful diet, several key supplements can also help to prevent type II diabetes, or prevent it from worsening.

Minerals

Chromium—Recent studies suggest that chromium can prevent type II diabetes, or insulin resistance. Chromium functions by increasing the activity of insulin, thus reducing the amount of insulin required to control blood-sugar levels. In one study, Richard Anderson, Ph.D., of the U.S.D.A. Human Nutrition Research Center (working with Chinese researchers at Beijing Hospital) tested the effect of chromium on adult patients in the early stages of type II diabetes. One group of patients was given 100 mcg.

of chromium picolinate twice daily, another group was given 500 mcg. of chromium picolinate twice daily, and a third group was given a placebo. After two months, the group receiving 100 mcg. daily showed a significant reduction in blood-sugar levels, a sign that their bodies were using insulin more effectively and, within four months, the group receiving the lower dosage also showed similar improvement. The placebo group showed virtually no change.

Earlier studies at the Vitamin and Mineral Nutrition Laboratory at the Beltsville Human Nutrition Research Center of the United States Department of Agriculture (1991) also suggested that insufficient dietary chromium can lead to impaired glucose tolerance, which can be alleviated by supplemental chromium.

Chromium is naturally found in many herbs and spices, such as turmeric and fenugreek which are used liberally in curries and chutney, but are not normally used in typical American cuisine. Unfortunately, few Americans get enough chromium from diet alone, which is why chromium supplements are so important.

Magnesium—Chronic magnesium deficiency can result in bone loss, high blood pressure, vascular disease, and abnormal blood-sugar metabolism. A study of forty-five diabetic and twelve normal children found children with insulin-dependent diabetes had lower levels of magnesium than normal children. These studies strongly suggest that low magnesium levels increase risk factors for diseases related to diabetes, and may even be a causative factor in the onset of the disease.

One of the increased risks diabetics face is hypertension. There is increasing evidence that magnesium deficiency may be a key factor leading to cardiovascular disease, including hypertension and atherosclerosis.

Studies show that magnesium can lower blood pressure, and improve the efficiency of insulin in older people. Good food sources of magnesium include bananas, apricots, curry powder, wheat bran, and whole grains.

Vitamins

Vitamin E—New research suggests vitamin E, a well-known antioxidant, may help people with type II diabetes better use insulin. In a study, twenty-five men and women, ten healthy subjects and fifteen with type II diabetes, took a glucose tolerance test before and after taking 900 milligrams of vitamin E per day for four months. At the end of the study, researchers found that the body-cell membranes of the diabetics who took vitamin E supplements were less insulin resistant, a sign that they were better able to metabolize sugar.

Vitamin B6—Vitamin B6 (pyridoxine) has been shown to help prevent *diabetic retinopathy*, a leading cause of blindness due to poor circulation.

Herbs

Garlic—We know that taking garlic supplements can lower blood cholesterol levels, but it may also have an antidiabetic effect. Garlic contains a compound called S-*allyl cysteine sulfoxide*, an amino acid that contains sulfur. Animal studies have shown that this compound significantly decreased blood-glucose and cholesterol levels.

Bilberry Extract—One of the most devastating effects of diabetes is blindness, which is the result of diabetic retinopathy, the destruction of small blood vessels which impair the blood flow to the eye. In a 1987 clinical study of forty diabetics, Italian researchers demonstrated a significant improvement in vision and measurable microcirculation resulting from compounds found in bilberry.

Personal Advice

Caution—If you are diabetic, do not attempt to self-medicate. Supplements can help, and may even reduce the need for other medication, but you must work with a knowledgeable physician or natural healer who can monitor your progress.

In a word, exercise!—A recent study surveyed 548 people with insulin-dependent diabetes mellitus. An analysis of their habits after six years revealed that the men who were more sedentary, expending less than 1,000 calories per week through exercise, were three times more likely to have died that the active men who used up more than 2,000 calories per week.

Research at the Human Nutrition Research Center on Aging at Tufts University, Boston, indicates that regular aerobic exercise can lower the risk of diabetes, even if no weight loss occurs in the process. A three-month study of eighteen older men and women who had above-normal glucose levels on glucose tolerance tests, showed that the eighteen volunteers cleared eleven percent more glucose from their blood after cycling on an exercise bike four days per week.

After twelve weeks, the exercise improved the ability of their cells to respond to insulin, allowing them to process the glucose more efficiently. The finding supports other research showing that exercise itself improves people's insulin sensitivity.

Isotonics, also known as strength training, weight training, or resistance training, builds muscle mass. Increased muscle mass also raises the body's metabolic rate, which means you burn extra calories. Greater muscle mass requires more calories than body fat to sustain itself, meaning you can lose fat without eating a lot less. Another benefit of greater muscle mass is that it decreases the risk for developing diabetes. The more muscle mass in the body, the less insulin it takes to get sugar, or glucose, out of the blood and into the tissues, where it's need for energy. Thus, the body is less likely to overuse insulin, which means the chance of developing adult-onset diabetes is lessened.

We already know that exercise, early detection of eye problems, low-fat and low-sugar diets, and a healthy lifestyle are important in controlling diabetic complications. Giving up smoking is another important lifestyle change in helping to prevent nerve disease. Your nerves are fed by small blood vessels. When these blood vessels are damaged, the nerves are deprived of oxygen and suffer damage. Smoking increases the risk of developing neuropathy and makes the condition worse once it begins, because smoking further damages blood vessels, which have already suffered damage from diabetes.

Alcohol has been shown to increase the risk of nerve disease in diabetics, and diabetics are encourage to drink in moderation, or not at all.

Since eye disease is a high risk factor for diabetics, and since antioxidants have been shown to reduce the risk of eye disease, it certainly makes sense for diabetics to increase their intake of antioxidant foods. Fruits and vegetables, especially dark-green vegetables, such as spinach, peppers, and broccoli are good sources; citrus fruits are a good source of vitamin C.

Diet tips—Slow-release nutrients, such as those found in legumes, can prevent a quick spike of blood sugar that can be difficult for the body to utilize. These legumes include beans, lentils, peas, and soybeans. Cutting back on simple carbohydrates (sugary snack foods) and loading up on dietary fiber, especially soluble fiber, is effective in normalizing mild to moderately elevated blood-glucose levels. A diet providing 50 to 60 percent of calories from carbohydrate and 20 to 35 grams of dietary fiber daily is typically recommended for diabetics, as well as the general population.

Earl's Rx

Chromium picolinate: One to three 200 mcg. tablets daily. (Up to 1000 mcg. have been given to adult onset diabetics. Check with your M.D.)

Magnesium: One 500 mg. tablet daily.

Vitamin E: One or two 400 IU capsules, dry form, daily.

Vitamin B6: Take 50–100 mg. daily.

Garlic: One raw, odorless garlic capsule daily.

Copper: Take 2–3 mg. tablet daily.

Ear Infections

These pesky and persistent infections can be the bane of childhood.

Hold the antibiotics!!! Reach for the *probiotics*. Natural immune-boosting remedies may be less toxic and more effective than antibiotics in treating ear infections.

E ar infections are one of the most common of all childhood diseases, and one of the trickiest to treat. Until recently, pediatricians would routinely prescribe antibiotics for ear infections, but those days are gone. The indiscriminate use of antibiotics has given rise to new and more virulent strains of antibiotic-resistant bacteria that are very difficult to beat. In fact, in many cases, antibiotics no longer work and may actually prolong the infection.

In a study of children with acute middle-ear infections, two Dutch physicians compared the effects of antibiotic treatment with the effects of no treatment at all. They studied 3,047 children; 1,680 were given antibiotics and 1,367 received no antibiotics. The results were astonishing: When antibiotics were begun on the first day of the infection, the frequency of recurrence was near three times higher than when no antibiotics are given! When antibiotics are begun after the eighth day, the rate of recurrence was less than one-and-a-half times higher. In other words, antibiotic therapy does not shorten the disease process, and may actually lengthen it. The researchers concluded that antibiotics should be reserved for instances in which complications are present, and that antibiotics are most effective when taking them is delayed and antibiotic therapy is infrequent.

In yet another study, antibiotics were shown to work in only 14 percent of children given antibiotics for middle-ear inflammation and fluid. As a result of this groundbreaking study, The American Academy of Pediatrics changed its guidelines for the treatment of ear infections, and now recommends that pediatricians wait up to four months before beginning any treatment to see if the ear infection heals on its own. If the inflammation and fluid does not clear up within that time, or if there is hearing loss, then doctors are advised to choose either antibiotics or surgery.

Here are some natural remedies that can help mother nature win the battle against ear infections.

Herbs

Echinacea—This flower, which grew abundantly throughout North America, was widely valued by Native Americans for its medicinal qualities. Early American physicians recognized the value of echinacea, especially in the treatment of infection. German studies from the 1950s through the 1980s confirmed the herb's remarkable healing and antiviral powers.

Echinacea fights infection with a natural antibiotic action derived from the roots or leaves of the plant. It has a milder effect on the body than a synthetic antibiotic, with few if any side effects. Unlike antibiotics, which work by destroying the invading organisms, echinacea stimulates the body's immune system, our natural defense against disease. It is a *probiotic*, that is, for life; it enhances our own ability to fight disease, strengthening our bodies in the process. A growing number of pediatricians are now turning to echinacea to treat children's colds and ear infections because of its anti-inflammatory and anti-infectious properties.

Garlic—Here's one remedy my grandmother used! Garlic oil, a popular folk remedy for earache, has recently made a comeback. A few drops of garlic oil from a garlic capsule gently applied to the ear with a cotton swab can help an earache. (Do not use eardrops if your child has surgically implanted ear tubes and do not put eardrops in the ear before visiting the doctor, because the oil will obstruct the doctor's view of the eardrum.)

Acidophilus—This "friendly bacteria," found in active yogurt cultures and sold in capsule and liquid form, can boost immune response, helping the body to ward off offending viruses and bacteria.

Personal Advice

A healthy immune system is best defense against infection. If your child is prone to ear infections, I recommend that you avoid giving your child cow's milk, which can often cause allergic reactions in children, and switch to soy milk. Studies show that soybean peptides (chains of amino acids) can boost the immune system. Consider adding soy products to your child's diet (tofu and soymilk are good choices).

Food allergies can cause congestion in the nose and throat, which can lead to ear infections. Check for food allergies and eliminate those foods that cause allergic reactions. Fresh fruit, especially citrus fruits, will add natural vitamin C to your child's diet. Green vegetables, plenty of exercise and fresh air, restful sleep (and enough sleep), all help to strengthen the immune system and keep your child in general good health.

Breastfeeding your baby will also offer powerful protection against ear infections, because you will pass your own disease-fighting antibodies on to your baby through breast milk. Researchers followed two groups of children up to age twenty-four months to determine how long the protective effect of breastfeeding lasts. Results indicate the risk of acute ear infections was significantly decreased until four months after breastfeeding was discontinued. As the months after weaning passed, the risk of infection gradually increased for infants who were not breastfed, with the risk reaching the same level for both groups within twelve months. The study concluded that the risk of acute ear infections in infants depends on both the number of months an infant is breastfed and the number of months that pass after breastfeeding is discontinued.

Earl's Rx

If your child has an acute ear infection, I recommend the following.

Echinacea: Take 500 mg., one to three times daily, for one week. Echinacea comes in capsules (for adults) and liquid for children. Give your child one to three droppersfull daily. Echinacea, which has a bitter flavor, can be mixed in a small amount of juice to make it more appealing to young palates.

Acidophilus: Take 1 teaspoon of acidophilus liquid daily. Keep acidophilus under refrigeration. You can mix acidophilus liquid with a small amount of juice to make it easier for your child to swallow. Acidophilus is also available in capsules, but I do not recommend capsules for small children. Some children past the age of ten, however, may be able to swallow capsules. If your child can take capsules, try giving him one capsule, two times daily, with food.

Fibromyalgia

Ninety percent of all people with fibromyalgia are women between the ages of twenty and fifty-five.

I hurt everywhere," is a common complaint of women suffering from *fibromyalgia,* a mysterious and potentially debilitating disorder, in which unspecified aches and pains are often accompanied by excessive fatigue. If fibromyalgia sounds similar to another problem that I discussed earlier, chronic fatigue syndrome, that is because the two disorders have much in common. There are some differences, however, notably that women with fibromyalgia may also experience other related problems, including irritable bowel syndrome, jaw pain or tenderness, insomnia, fatigue, premenstrual syndrome, feelings of feverishness and chills without elevated temperatures, and even chest pain.

Since fibromyalgia mimics so many other disorders, it is often difficult to make a definitive diagnosis. Recently, the American College of Rheumatology established guidelines to help physicians distinguish a true case of fibromyalgia from other medical problems. According to these guidelines, in order to diagnose fibromyalgia, a patient must have widespread aches and pains in at least eleven of eighteen standard tender points. These points are located in the hip, ankle, knees, upper chest, jaw, neck, upper and lower back, elbow, and wrist. Although these tender points may cause substantial pain, what is particularly mystifying about this problem is that medical tests will not show any physical abnormalities causing the pain.

Very often, however, fibromyalgia is a diagnosis of exclusion. When all other obvious ailments are ruled out, and no other cause can be found, such as arthritis, other connective-tissue diseases, or even a sluggish thyroid (which could cause fatigue) a diagnosis of fibromyalgia may be considered.

Some researchers suspect that fibromyalgia may be triggered by an undetected viral infection. In fact, several studies have revealed that certain components of the immune system behave abnormally with patients suspected of having fibromyalgia, and there are signs of changes in immune function which may indicate that the immune system is waging a low-grade battle against an infectious agent. Therefore, strengthening the immune system may be an important factor in relieving symptoms. (See "Immune Weakness," p. 165.)

Researchers are also exploring the possibility that fibromyalgia may be the result of an underlying sleep disorder. Electroencephalographic (EEG) studies have shown that those patients with disturbed sleep patterns also exhibit many of the symptoms of fibromyalgia. Although it is not clear whether the disturbed sleep patterns cause fibromyalgia, or whether the symptoms of the disorder cause the disturbed sleep patterns, researchers are hopeful that this clue will lead to better treatment.

A recent study of the levels of neural hormones (chemicals that carry messages between the brain and central nervous system) showed some evidence that women who have fibromyalgia have lower than normal levels of chemicals that are vital to muscle repair and are released by the liver in response to growth hormone. Although we don't understand the precise mechanism, this could be a factor that leads to fibromyalgia.

Since clinically depressed patients also have immune problems similar to people with fibromyalgia, there may be a connection between depression, the immune system, and this puzzling disorder.

Unfortunately, there is no simple cure for the problem and, for most patients, the solution is often careful management of their symptoms.

Herbs

Capsaicin—Hot-pepper cream, which has been used successfully to treat arthritis, shows promise as a treatment for the pain of fibromyalgia. Capsaicin is one of the compounds that makes chili pepper hot. In a recent double-blind trial at the Department of Medicine of the Medical College of Wisconsin, forty-five patients with primary fibromyalgia rubbed either capsaicin cream or a placebo ointment into aching points on one side of the body four times a day for four weeks. The untreated side of the body served as a control.

At the end of four weeks, the patients who used capsaicin reported less pain on both sides of the body (treated and untreated), along with an increase in grip strength, than those who received the placebo.

Evening primrose oil—This herb is often used to treat rheumatoid arthritis or the inflammation of the soft tissue of the joints. It may relieve some of the joint pain associated with fibromyalgia.

Antioxidants—Antioxidants, such as vitamin E and coenzyme Q10, can help reduce inflammation, and will protect against free-radical damage, which is believed to exacerbate this condition.

Personal Advice

Exercise is absolutely vital for those suffering from the symptoms of fibromyalgia, in order to increase cardiovascular capacity and improve muscle tone. Low-impact exercise such as swimming, bicycling, stretching, walking, and low-impact aerobics are recommended. You will probably suffer more pain during the first few weeks of an exercise program, but it's worth it, because as your muscles become conditioned, pain eases.

People with fibromyalgia must be particularly vigilant about controlling stress, since women often report that symptoms worsen during periods of emotional crises. Inasmuch as the onset of the disease is often precipitated by periods of great stress, such as divorce, job change, moving, or a death in the family, stress management may play a key role in restoring good health.

Yoga, acupressure, message therapy, biofeedback, and other stress relievers can help. Because many doctors either do not recognize the disorder, or are at a loss as to how to treat it, you must assume responsibility for managing your illness. Demand extensive tests to rule out other conditions, seek out a physician who has experience dealing with muscle pain, and investigate ways to achieve sound sleep. (See "Sleep Disorders," p. 242.) Ask your physician or natural healer for natural ways to control depression and stress.)

A positive outlook is extremely important, since fibromyalgia is not fatal and usually doesn't get worse. Depression only leads to a vicious cycle of pain, disturbed sleep, fatigue, then more depression.

Avoid caffeine; it can promote insomnia and can make you feel jittery, which will only make your condition worse. Examples would be soft drinks, colas, coffee, tea, chocolate, and pain relievers, either over-the-counter or by prescription.

Earl's Rx

Fibromyalgia is difficult to treat, but the following supplements may help.

Coenzyme Q10: Take one 30–60 mg capsule daily. (This potent antioxidant may help joint pain.)

Vitamin E: One 400–800 IU capsule in dry form, taken with food.

Grapeseed and green-tea extract (in combination tablets): Take one tablet, three times daily.

Evening primrose oil: One 500 mg. capsule, up to three times daily.

Gallstones

Removal of the gallbladder is the fifth most-common operation performed in the U.S.

A change in diet and lifestyle, and the right supplements will enable many people to manage gallbladder problems without surgery.

The gallbladder is a small, pear-shaped sac that stores *bile,* a substance secreted by the liver which aids in the digestion of fats and is eventually discharged into the small intestine. *Gallstones* are solid masses that form in the gallbladder or bile ducts. There are three types of gallstones: combination stones consisting of calcium, bile, cholesterol, and other substances; stones of pure cholesterol; and stones of pure bile. Depending on the size and type of gallstones, the gallbladder can become infected and inflamed, which can be quite painful and, in some cases, the gallbladder will have to surgically removed.

The risk factors for gallbladder disease include a high-fat, high-cholesterol diet, alcohol-related liver disease, chronic inflammations of the liver or gallbladder, food allergies, genetic predisposition, and parasite infections.

Depending on the type of gallstones, various drugs may be prescribed to shrink the stones. In some cases, ultrasound waves may be used to dissolve the stones without surgery. In this treatment, sonic waves bombard the stones so that they are more readily broken down. This non-invasive treatment is safe, but does not prevent the formation of future gallstones.

A chronic gallbladder problem can cause great discomfort, including gasiness, nausea, and abdominal cramps. If possible, the best approach is to try to prevent the problem from occurring in the first place. Here are some supplements that can help.

Fat Busters

Lecithin—*Lecithin* is a phospholipid, that is, a substance produced by the liver that is involved in the metabolism of fat. Available as a supplement, lecithin is often prescribed by both physicians and natural healers to reduce the size of cholesterol gallstones. Anyone with a tendency to develop gallstones should take supplemental lecithin daily.

Taurine—This amino acid, which is found in bile salts, helps increase bile formation and excretion. Since bile is essential for the breakdown of fats and lipids, a lack of this important substance can result in a buildup of cholesterol. Women's bodies make less taurine than do men's, which may explain why women have a twice the risk for developing cholesterol gallstones.

Herbs

Milk thistle—This herb contains a compound called *silymarin*, an antioxidant that can protect the liver from oxidative damage due to free radicals. Milk thistle can also stimulate the growth of new liver cells to replace old, damaged cells. Since healthy liver function is vital to healthy gallbladder function, milk thistle is an important addition to the arsenal of herbs used to relieve gallbladder disorders. In addition, milk thistle may help prevent or treat gallstones directly by increasing the solubility of the bile secreted by the gallbladder, enabling it to pass more quickly through the body.

Peppermint—This herb has been used for centuries as a treatment for digestive disorders, including excessive gasiness, which is one symptom of gallstones. Peppermint is now used in various herbal formulas designed to dissolve gallstones.

Turmeric—This spice, which gives curry powder its characteristic yellow color, is used as a treatment for gallstones, usually in combination with other herbs such as milk thistle and peppermint. Indian healers have known of its medicinal value for centuries and used it to preserve food (it has an antibacterial component) and to treat obesity. Researchers now know that turmeric has a beneficial effect on the liver, stimulating the flow of bile, which helps break down dietary fats, which in turn protects and treats disorders of the gallbladder.

Dandelion—This weed is a natural diuretic and digestive aid, rich in lecithin and potassium, which enhance liver and gallbladder function.

Personal Advice

Diet tips—Gallstones are associated with the so-called western diet, which is high in refined carbohydrates and fat and low in fiber. If you suffer from chronic gallbladder inflammation, your best bet is to switch to a very low-fat diet. For some people, this may mean eliminating meat and animal products and adopting a vegetarian diet. In all cases, a diet high in water-soluble fibers (found in vegetables, fruits, pectin, and oat bran) is extremely important in the prevention as well as the reversal of most gallstones. Decrease the amount of sugar and refined carbohydrates and try eating more frequent small meals during the course of the day, avoiding that large meal that is usually eaten at the end of the day.

Food allergies have been known to trigger gallbladder inflammation. Consult a physician to determine if certain foods are causing your discomfort.

Earl's Rx

Lecithin granules (98 % pure): One tablespoon two to three times daily.

Taurine: One 250 mg. capsule up to two times daily, in-between meals.

Milk thistle: One to three capsules daily.

Combination supplement for gallbladder health: I recommend a combination herbal formula, that is, one capsule containing peppermint, dandelion, and turmeric. Several commercial brands are available at natural-food stores. Take one to three capsules daily.

Gastrointestinal Disorders

GI disorders are a virtual epidemic in the United States—diet is a major culprit.

The cure? A change in diet and lifestyle.

The gastrointestinal tract—which begins at the mouth and ends at the rectum—is a 30-foot tube through which the food we eat is broken down, so that it can be utilized by the body and the waste products eliminated. The digestion of food is critical to sustain life. From food, we get the energy we need to run every bodily system. In the United States, disorders of the GI tract are as common as the cold and, like the common cold, natural remedies are often more effective for GI problems than drugs.

Constipation—The most common chronic GI problem is constipation, characterized by stool that is difficult to pass, or bowel movements too infrequent for comfort. Constipation is not just uncomfortable, but can promote hemorrhoids, a type of varicose vein which can be extremely painful. (See page 267.) The primary cause of constipation is a diet high in refined carbohydrates and low in fiber. Ideally, we should consume 20–40 grams of fiber daily, but few Americans actually do. Fiber is found in whole grains, fruits and vegetables; it is absent from products made with white flour, as well as the types of processed and convenience foods that are the mainstay of the American diet. The two types of fiber, soluble and insoluble, are of equal importance. Insoluble fiber softens and bulks waste so that it moves quickly through the colon, the last stop on the GI tract before it is eliminated from the body. Soluble fiber binds with bile, a product produced by the liver which is essential for the absorption of fat, and is excreted in the feces. Since excess bile can result in bile stones, it is important to move it through the body as quickly as possible. Soluble fiber can also help to lower cholesterol.

Fiber not only can prevent constipation, but may prevent a much greater problem—colon cancer. Studies have shown a direct link between the rate of colon cancer and the amount of fiber in the diet. In fact, in countries where fiber is consumed in high quantities, colon cancer is a rarity. Why? The theory is, the faster food moves through the GI

127

tract, the less exposure there is to pesticides and other carcinogens that can be found in food.

Good sources of insoluble fiber include celery, legumes, leafy green vegetables, and whole grains.

Good sources of soluble fiber include apples, bananas, oat bran, and strawberries.

Drinking eight to ten glasses of filtered water daily is essential for proper digestion and can prevent constipation. A lack of exercise is also a likely cause of constipation, particularly for people who have sedentary jobs. A brisk walk daily can help keep your digestive juices flowing and your body working at its best. In addition, certain commonly prescribed medications such as diuretics, painkillers, and tranquilizers, can cause constipation. If you are taking any drugs on a regular basis and have a problem with constipation, check with your physician to see if your medication could be the cause.

Many Americans turn to laxatives to help them with constipation, a practice that I do not recommend. Laxatives can not only become habit-forming, but can sap your body of important nutrients. I prefer that people get their fiber through food; however, if you simply cannot eat enough fiber-rich foods, some supplements may be helpful.

Diarrhea—Diarrhea is the opposite of constipation; it is characterized by stool that is too watery or occurs too frequently. Diarrhea is most often caused by a mild bacterial or viral infection, but it can also be due to something more serious, such as a parasite. In some cases, a sudden increase in foods containing a high amount of insoluble fiber can cause the runs. In most cases, diarrhea simply clears up on its own; however, due to the loss of fluid and important minerals, it can leave you feeling tired and drained. If you have diarrhea, it is essential to replenish the lost fluids by drinking lots of clear broth, filtered water, apple juice, and herbal tea, as well as minerals, particularly potassium.

Pectin, a form of soluble fiber found in fruits and vegetables, can also help to reduce diarrhea by absorbing water and important minerals in the bowel. Foods rich in pectin include apples, carrots, rice, and bananas; it is also available in capsules.

Blueberries are an excellent food to eat when you have diarrhea. They are not only rich in pectin, but contain compounds called *anthocyanosides,* which have a mild antibiotic action that can help to knock out the infection that may be causing the problem.

Acidophilus, which is found in active yogurt cultures, is an excellent way to restore the normal bacterial balance in your gut, and can prevent the kind of infections that can lead to diarrhea.

Diverticulosis—Half of all people over age sixty have diverticulosis, a condition characterized by the presence of tiny saclike pouches called *diverticula* in the wall of the colon. The major risk factor for diverticulosis is a history of chronic constipation. Clearly, to prevent this problem from occurring in the first place, the key is to prevent constipation. Once you have diverticulosis, it is even more important to maintain regular bowel movements. Constipation can cause the diverticula to become inflamed, and that can cause a more serious condition called *diverticulitis,* which requires immediate medical care and can lead to intestinal obstruction.

The usual treatment for diverticulosis is a high fiber diet, which will prevent the kind of inflammation that can lead to the more serious diverticulitis. Diverticulitis is treated quite differently, however, usually with antibiotics and a low-fat diet.

Earl's Rx

Psyllium (Constipation and Diverticulosis): Add between a teaspoon and a tablespoon of psyllium powder to water or juice daily and follow with two glasses of water. (Although it is rare, psyllium can cause an allergic reaction in some people. If you are allergic to different foods, check with your physician or natural healer before using psyllium.)

Pectin (Diarrhea): Increase your intake of pectin: Eat a grated raw carrot or grated apple with skin. Pectin is also available in capsules. Take two capsules three times daily.

Potassium: One 99 mg. tablet three times daily.

For general GI health: One tablespoon of acidophilus liquid three times daily between meals, or take two capsules three times daily between meals.

Gout

Over 2 million Americans suffer the excruciating pain and swelling of gout.

More than 95 percent of gout sufferers are men over the age of thirty.

The number of Americans with this disorder has doubled over the past thirty years.

G out used to be a disease associated with affluence: If you had gout, it was a sign that you ate too much of the wrong kinds of food. In reality, gout is a form of arthritis caused by an excess amount of uric acid, a byproduct of a substance called *purine,* found in certain types of foods including meat, anchovies, asparagus, chicken, and mushrooms. A defect in the way uric acid is broken down by the body causes an excess of uric acid and urates (uric-acid salts) to accumulate in the bloodstream and the joints. This results in the destruction of the joints and deposits of salt in the skin and cartilage, especially of the big toe. The excess of uric-acid salts also damages the kidneys, which can cause kidney stones. You don't have to be a glutton to get this disease; it is caused by a simple error in metabolism and, for some people, just a small amount of the wrong food will trigger an attack.

The typical treatment for gout involves the prescription of drugs (allopurinol) that increase the excretion of uric acid, or which slow the formation of uric acid salts. If you have severe gout, allopurinol can help relieve your symptoms. Here are some other supplements and foods that can help to prevent a flare-up.

Herbs

Cherry Juice—Cherries can lower uric-acid levels, and cherry juice is used in Europe as a bona fide treatment for gout. Other helpful fruits include hawthorn berries, blueberries, juniper berries, and other dark-red-blue berries. These berries are rich in anthocyanidin and proanthocyanidin, believed to help normalize uric acid levels.

Grapeseed—Grapeseed contains bioflavonoids, substances which give fruits their color. Bioflavonoids work with vitamin C to prevent the destruction of collagen, which can exacerbate arthritic symptoms.

Celery juice—This juice is an excellent diuretic that promotes the flow of urine through the kidneys and may relieve the symptoms of gout.

Personal advice

Avoiding the wrong foods can go a long way in preventing gout. Foods high in purine should be off limits: they include dried legumes, liver, mackerel, sardines, shrimp, sweetbreads, asparagus, bran, cauliflower, eel, saltwater fish, legumes, meat, spinach, and whole grains. Some foods may be more irritating than others. Try to keep a food diary to see which foods seem to trigger the worst symptoms.

Reduce the amount of overall protein you consume each day. Drink lots of fluids to flush uric acid from your body and prevent kidney stones, and avoid excessive alcohol.

Overweight may exacerbate gout; lose weight if you need to, but moderation is the key. Losing weight *too* fast may actually increase uric acid levels. Healthy eating with an emphasis on low-fat, low-sugar food, and exercise will help maintain proper weight.

Earl's Rx

Drink one glass of cherry juice up to three times daily, and try the following supplements.

Grapeseed extract: Take 100 mg. three times daily.

Vitamin B-complex: One 50 mg. tablet or capsule two to three times daily, with food.

Vitamin B6: One 50 mg. tablet three times daily.

Multiple antioxidant: Look for a combination containing alpha and betacarotene, superoxide dismutase, vitamins C, E, and selenium. Take two to three daily.

Headache

Approximately 40 million Americans seek medical help for headaches every year.

8 to 10 percent of all headaches treated by physicians are migraine headaches.

Approximately 60 percent of all migraine sufferers are women.

Next to the common cold, headaches are probably the most prevalent of all health problems. Nearly everyone has experienced the relentless throb or dull ache characteristic of most headaches and, for many, the symptoms are far worse. For an unlucky few, the pain can be excrutiating.

Not all headaches are the same. Headaches generally fall into four different categories: *tension headache, cluster headache, traction and inflammatory headache,* and *migraine headache.* However, experts are learning that headaches are difficult to characterize and the symptoms of one type of headache often overlap with symptoms of other kinds of head pain.

The most common brand of headache is the tension headache, which often feels like the head is being squeezed by a tight band. Muscle spasm brought on by tension is thought to cause this type of headache. Other possible causes of tension headache include anger, frustration, muscle strain from physical work, poor posture, eyestrain, and grinding the teeth.

Cluster headaches most often occur in men. This type of headache produces short, severe attacks of excruciating pain centered over one eye. Attacks may recur in cluster headaches many times a day for several months, and then disappear for months at a time. Treatment can be managed but there is no known cure.

Traction and inflammatory headaches are symptoms of other, more serious disorders, ranging from stroke to sinus infection.

The most debilitating headache is probably the migraine. If you feel exhausted and slightly dizzy, if the sight and smell of food nauseates you, if loud noise is unbearable and bright light is painful, if your head pounds, and you can't concentrate, you probably have a migraine.

Migraine is also characterized by visual disturbances or what is called an aura that many patients experience before the pain begins, which typically include visions of flashing lights or geometric designs.

Research scientists are unclear about the precise cause of migraine headaches, which makes treatment complicated, but most researchers agree all migraine headaches involve blood-flow changes to the brain.

What can trigger a migraine headache? There are many possibilities, ranging from food allergies to chemical exposure, either at home or in the workplace. It may require some real detective work to determine what triggers your headache, but it is possible. First, look to what you are eating. Is it red wine, chocolate, nuts, beans, fermented foods like yogurt, Chinese food, shellfish, hot dogs, cold cuts, alcohol, coffee, colas, or cheese? These foods and others contain chemical substances such as tyramine, nitrates, monosodium glutamate, or caffeine, which constrict or dilate arteries. The next step is to look to your environment. Do certain smells such as found in solvents, paints, or perfumes trigger the attack? Do bright or flickering lights bring on a headache?

Can severe stress trigger a migraine attack? Perhaps. Some researchers believe that stress affects certain chemicals in the brain called *neurotransmitters*. Signals carried by these neurotransmitters may cause the blood vessels of the head to relax, and the area around them to become inflamed. The inflammation irritates the endings of a complex nerve called the *trigeminal nerve*, which in turn causes the throbbing pain of migraine.

Researchers also believe an excess or deficiency of brain chemicals plays a part. These chemicals include norepinephrine, serotonin, prostaglandins, and endorphins, all of which are the brain's own opiate substances. Coincidentally, patients suffering from depression, sleep disorders, and drug abuse show a deficiency of some of these same chemicals, suggesting either a genetic propensity for migraine and other types of headache, or a family dysfunction that tends to perpetuate itself from generation to generation. For many people the headache doesn't occur during stressful times, but *after* a period of high pressure. The explanation for this phenomenon is that headaches can be caused by an initial constriction of blood vessels to the brain, then when the person relaxes, the vessels suddenly dilate, causing a cycle of pain: the pain causes distress, the distress causes the vessels to constrict once more, and the patient can't seem to get out of the headache cycle.

Since three times as many women as men suffer from migraine, researchers believe fluctuating female hormones may play a role in causing headaches. Sixty percent of women headache sufferers report severe headaches shortly before, during, or just after, their period. Further credence is given to the theory of hormone-induced headache by the fact that migraines tend to subside during pregnancy, disappear after menopause, and recur when a women begins estrogen replacement therapy.

Head pain is nothing new—it has plagued civilization throughout history and there have probably been thousands of remedies that have been tried, some successfully, some not. For example, for thousands of years the Chinese have used acupuncture to relieve head pain and still do. They were light years ahead of medieval physicians who used cathartics and bloodletting to treat migraines, neither of which is believed to have had any therapuetic benefit. The pre-Columbian Incas of Peru and ancient Egyptians drilled holes in the skull to release the evil spirits they believed caused the problem and I suspect even if their patients survived the ordeal, their heads hurt even more after the treatment than before!

Today, treating headaches is very big business. Americans spend more than 400 million dollars a year on over-the-counter painkillers, and people with recurring headaches often become addicted to the drugs. There are many drugs, prescription and over-the-counter, available to treat headaches; they are not effective for everyone and some have significant side effects. Even a drug as simple as aspirin can irritate the stomach, high doses of acetaminophen can cause kidney problems, and, in large amounts, ibuprofen can also cause stomach trouble. Worse, large and frequent does of analgesics can lead to "rebound" headaches. That is, when the patient stops taking the drugs, the pain returns with even greater intensity and stronger medication is needed for relief. That is why I feel that, whenever possible, it is advisable to treat headaches with natural remedies, which in most cases are kinder and gentler to the body.

A word of advice before you self-medicate: If headache pain persists for more than a few days, check with your physician or natural healer. It could be a symptom of another problem. In some cases, these natural remedies may not work; don't suffer in silence. Ask for help!

Herbs

White willow bark—I love this herb! It's gentle, but it can be very effective. The analgesic properties of white willow bark have been known throughout the ages. Ancient Egyptian, Assyrian, and Greek physicians and Native Americans used it for headache. *Salicylic acid,* the compound from which aspirin was synthesized, was first derived from willow bark in 1838. In addition, in its natural state white willow bark yields other components that enhance its analgesic properties.

Ginger—I never take a trip without packing a few ginger capsules! This herb, which is excellent for motion sickness, may help prevent and ease effects of migraine headache without any side effects. Ginger root is usually used to soothe an upset stomach, and is wonderful for controlling that sick, nauseated feeling that accompanies a migraine.

Feverfew—This herb is a member of the sunflower family and has been used for centuries for the treatment of migraine and inflammatory disease, such as arthritis. This herb enhances the secretion of two neurotransmitters, histamine and serotonin.

In a six-month double-blind study at London Migraine Clinic, patients who had been previously helped by eating feverfew were given a replacement placebo instead. Another group of migraine patients were given feverfew. The placebo group suffered a significant increase in the frequency and severity of headache, nausea, and vomiting. In contrast, the patients taking feverfew reported a noticeable decline of those symptoms. Two patients in the placebo group had to withdraw from the study because of their recurring migraine headaches.

In another double blind study at the University of Nottingham, seventy-two patients were randomly given either a placebo or feverfew daily. After four months patients had their supplements switched and tests were continued for another four months. Those treated with feverfew had a 24 percent reduction in the number of migraine episodes, and those who continued to have headaches noticed a significant decrease in the severity and duration of attacks. Results of these studies were published in the British medical journal *Lancet*.

Capsaicin—Capsaicin, a compound found in hot chili peppers, causes nerve fibers to release a neurotransmitter (called *substance P*) that carries messages to the brain. Repeated contact with capsaicin depletes the nerve chemical resulting in fewer pain messages reaching the brain.

Preliminary studies in the Netherlands and Norway have shown that repeated nasal-spray applications of capsaicin prevented the occurrence and severity of cluster headache attacks. Patients received either capsaicin or a placebo in the nostril that corresponded to the side of the head where the pain was localized.

There was a significant decrease in headache severity in the capsaicin group, but not in the placebo group.

Minerals

Magnesium—Too little magnesium has also been implicated a cause of headaches, particularly migraines. A study in the *Family Practice News* (August 15, 1993) reported low magnesium levels in thirteen of thirty-two patients with migraine. Magnesium supplements daily may reduce migraine incidence in individuals prone to headaches.

Zinc—Excess copper and too little zinc may cause migraines. Copper stimulates activity of *vasoactive amines,* chemicals that influence the size of blood vessels. Too much activity can trigger a migraine. Small amounts of zinc supplements may help keep copper levels down.

Aromatherapy

Soothing smells can quell an angry headache. External applications of mixed essential oils have long been used for relieving stress and headaches. These preparations usually contain peppermint, eucalyptus, and other oils, and are rubbed on the temples and forehead to relieve pain. Researchers at Germany's Neurological Clinic of the University of Kiel conducted a double-blind trial of peppermint and eucalyptus oils for headache pain. Thirty-two healthy subjects tried different preparations containing a placebo with traces of essential oils, or preparations containing both peppermint and eucalyptus oils, or preparations containing one or the other of the oils. The preparation containing nearly pure peppermint oil was the most effective.

Vitamins

What you eat may affect your ability to withstand pain. Here's why. In recent years, researchers have discovered that the body produces its own natural pain killers, called *endorphins.* Diets high in certain nutrients, notably choline, may supply the raw ingredients for these chemicals. Choline is found in the B vitamins, especially B1, B2, B6, and in vitamin E.

Personal Advice

Relieve stress—I know this is easier said than done, but keeping a handle on stress can go a long way in preventing headaches in the first place. Practice relaxation techniques, such as meditation and yoga. Exercise is also an excellent stress buster.

Avoid food triggers—Since certain foods are known to trigger migraine, you must make a real effort to find out which foods affect you. This may be as simple as keeping a record of everything you eat every day for several months, then recording the times and duration of migraine attacks. Compare your food chart with your headache chart and you may have the answer! A more drastic solution is to go on an elimination diet where you slowly introduce different foods into your diet daily. Then, when a particular food triggers an attack it can be quickly eliminated from the diet.

Headbands—Special headbands that can help relieve the symptoms of migraines are sold at pharmacies. Simply place the headband on your forehead and pull tightly; this reduces the blood flow to the brain temporarily and can reduce inflammation and pain. Some people find that if they use this band in the very early stages of a migraine, they can hold the headache at bay.

Earl's Rx

If you have a headache, or are prone to them, these supplements should help.

If you have a headache:

Ginger: Two ginger capsules three times daily to relieve nausea that may accompany a headache.

White willow bark: One or two 500 mg. capsules, up to three times daily.

To prevent a headache:

Gingko biloba: Two 60 mg. capsules or tablets, twice daily.

Magnesium: Take 500 mg. of chelated magnesium daily.

Zinc: One 15–50 mg. tablet or capsule daily.

Vitamin B complex: One 50–150 mg. capsule daily.

Hearing Loss

Hearing loss can begin early in life, but seems to worsen with age.

Good lifetime nutrition may help prevent age-related hearing loss.

You may think of the ear as the organ that is primarily responsible for hearing but, in fact, the ear has two important jobs in the body. Of course, it is the instrument which transmits sound, but it is also the organ that is responsible for helping us to maintain our balance. The human ear consists of three parts: the outer, middle, and inner portions. The outer ear is the part we can see; the middle ear is an air-filled chamber containing the eardrum, which serves to receive and amplify sound waves; and the inner ear contains the sensory receptors for hearing, which are enclosed in a fluid-filled chamber called the *cochlea*. It is in the inner ear in which sound waves in the air are converted to nerve impulses that are relayed to the brain, where they are interpreted as sound.

The innermost part of the ear maintains the body's balance. When we change the position of our head or body, the inner ear transmits nerve impulses to the brain, which help to restore our equilibrium.

Diseases of the ear include infection, tinnitus (ringing in the ear), rupture of the eardrum, Meniere's disease (vertigo), and various types of deafness.

Age-related decline in hearing can begin at around age twenty, when there is a gradual loss in high-frequency hearing. However, the loss is usually so minimal that it is hardly noticeable; it usually isn't until around age sixty that hearing loss becomes apparent. That's when there may be a loss of middle- and low-frequency sounds, making it more difficult to understand speech.

Hearing loss can be exacerbated by chronic exposure to loud noises, which can cause damage to the nerves. Atherosclerosis can also cause hearing loss by preventing the flow of blood and nutrients to the ear, which can also damage the delicate inner ear apparatus.

Clearly, two primary ways to prevent major hearing loss are to avoid excess exposure to loud noise, and to prevent cardiovascular disease.

Herbs

Ginkgo biloba—The ginkgo biloba tree predates the Ice Age, and the trees are believed capable of living two thousand to four thousand years. It's no wonder, then, that generations of healers from Asia to Europe have looked to the ginkgo for help in treating dozens of different diseases.

Modern science has not overlooked this miracle herb. Years of scientific research have shown that gingko leaves contain two major flavonoids (quercetin and kampferol), in addition to many other components that have a positive effect on circulation.

Ginkgo biloba extract (GBx) works to improve hearing loss by increasing the flow of blood to the ear. Screening trials in humans using ginkgo extract have shown promising results for hearing loss that is a consequence of head injury, exposure to loud noise, or circulatory problems.

Minerals

Magnesium—It has been well-documented that chronic exposure to loud noise can cause considerable hearing loss, regardless of age. In fact, many young people who serve in the military suffer hearing loss because of exposure to explosions in battlefield conditions. A simple mineral may help to prevent some of this damage. Researchers evaluated three hundred healthy young recruits with normal hearing who underwent two months of basic military training during which they were exposed to repeated high levels of noise. In this study, some of the recruits were given daily magnesium supplements, and some received a placebo. Noise-induced damage was more severe in the placebo group than the magnesium group.

Vitamins

B12—Adequate levels of vitamin B12 may help protect the hearing of people who are continually exposed to loud noise. Researchers in Israel examined a group of 113 whose average age was thirty-nine years. Fifty-seven of the men had tinnitus as well as measurable hearing loss caused by ear-splitting work environments. Another twenty-nine had some hearing loss, and twenty-seven had normal hearing.

Measurements of B12 levels in the hearing-impaired men showed nearly half the men with tinnitus and hearing loss were deficient in the vitamin, while only 19 percent of those with normal hearing were low in the nutrient. Researchers believe that B12 supplements probably would not help once the damage was done, but that lifetime good nutrition, which includes adequate B12, might prevent the damage. Good sources of B12 include lean meat, poultry, fish, shellfish, and low-fat dairy foods.

Personal Advice

Hearing loss is a growing problem that seems to be affecting people at younger and younger ages. Not so coincidentally, this finding correlates with the invention of headphones and sophisticated sound systems. In other words, your mother was right! Listening to music at ear-shattering decibel levels could cause permanent deafness.

Normal speech is usually around 65 to 70 decibels—the level at which noise is dangerous is 85 to 90 decibels. Exposure to loud noises, whether it is in the workplace (drills, motors, machinery), in the home, (lawn mowers, vacuum cleaners), or at play (music, fireworks, crowded sports events), could be detrimental to your hearing health. If you cannot avoid loud noises in your work or play, use protective headphones, or earplugs.

Good cardiovascular health is vital to keeping the blood flowing to the head. Exercise, eating well-balanced meals, reducing high blood pressure, and getting enough restful sleep all help to maintain good overall health, which will lessen the degree of hearing loss as you age.

Earl's Rx

These three supplements can help you to maintain good hearing.

Gingko biloba: One 60 mg. capsule or tablet, three times daily.

Magnesium: One 500 mg. tablet daily.

Vitamin B12: One 800–1200 mcg. capsule daily, sublingual form preferred.

Heart Disease

Heart disease has been the number-one killer in the United States since 1900.

One in six men and one in eight women age forty-five and over have had a heart attack or stroke.

Numerous studies have shown that change in diet and lifestyle can have a dramatic effect on reducing risk and even *reversing* heart disease.

Nearly two decades ago, when I first began writing about the role vitamins and other supplements play in the prevention of disease, the most common treatment for heart disease was bypass surgery. The mere suggestion that heart disease could be prevented and maybe surgery wasn't the panacea that it was cracked up to be, was considered to be nothing short of heresy. Those of us who recommended modest changes in diet and lifestyle along with key supplements as a method of keeping heart disease at bay were considered way out, while those who advocated risky and often unsuccessful open-heart surgery were considered sensible and mainstream.

Millions of heart operations later, the medical establishment has changed its tune. Thankfully, physicians today are becoming increasingly open-minded about using supplements instead of surgery, and about recommending diet, exercise, and stress reduction as part of their treatment plan.

The more we learn about heart disease, the more we see that, in many cases, it is completely preventable and that the best approach is to prevent the underlying problems that allow heart disease to take hold in the first place.

The heart is a muscle that maintains blood flow in the circulatory system. In order for blood to flow freely throughout the body, the *arteries* and *capillaries* (the hoses through which blood travels) must remain clear. Coronary artery disease or *atherosclerosis,* the most common cause of heart disease, occurs when the blood vessels become clogged with *plaque,* a thick, yellowish waxy substance that can build up and eventually obstruct blood flow. If the blood flow to the heart is cut off by plaque deposits, it will result in a heart attack. Strokes are usually caused by fat-clogged arteries that cut off the supply of blood to the brain.

What causes plaque? Plaque consists of a variety of cells including *cholesterol,* a fat or lipid that is primarily produced by the liver. Although cholesterol may appear to be the culprit in the heart-disease story, it is not that simple. In fact, there are two types of cholesterol, and one kind is actually good for you. The good cholesterol, *high density lipoprotein* (HDL), actually helps clean out the arteries by removing cholesterol from the blood and returning it to the liver where it can be broken down. The bad cholesterol, *low density lipoprotein,* (LDL) transports cholesterol from the liver to the millions of cells in the body. Although our bodies need both kinds of cholesterol to function properly, too much of either type of cholesterol can cause major problems.

Cholesterol is found in food, primarily dairy products and meat, but it is not enough to simply avoid foods high in cholesterol, since cholesterol is also produced in the body from fat found in food. (Fat contains one or more fatty acids. Some of these fatty acids are produced by the body, but some must be obtained through food.) Not all fat is the same however, and some types of fat can be more heart-healthy than others. For example, it is wise to limit your intake of saturated fat, which is found in animal products, because it is converted into cholesterol in the body. On the other hand, polyunsaturated fat and monounsaturated fat, both found in plant food and abundant in vegetable oil, can actually be beneficial and help to lower cholesterol. Not all forms of polyunsaturated fat are good, however, and some can actually be harmful. For example, hydrogenated vegetable oil, the type used in hard margarine, can also increase cholesterol levels. As a rule, stick to soft margarine and heart-healthy oils such as olive or safflower oil.

No more than 20 percent of your total daily caloric intake should come from fat of any kind, but this doesn't mean that you should eliminate fat altogether. Not at all. Surprisingly, eating too little fat may be as damaging as eating too much. Preliminary studies by researchers from the Boston University School of Medicine show that a very low-fat diet may in itself touch off heart disease. They found that a major risk factor was an insufficient intake of two polyunsaturated fats that are essential to human nutrition.

These essential fatty acids, *linoleic acid* and *linolenic acid,* are unsaturated fats that cannot be manufactured by the body and must be consumed in the diet. They are plentiful in foods like soybeans, various nuts and seeds, and green leafy vegetables—not exactly staples of the typical American meat-and-potatoes diet. Linoleic acid, an omega-6 fatty acid, is especially prominent in safflower oil, corn oil, cottonseed oil, and soybean oil. Linolenic acid, found in soybean and canola oil, flaxseed and purslane, is an omega-3 fatty acid like those in fish oils. Other studies suggest that an increase of omega-3 fatty acids found in fish oil are associated with a reduced risk of blood clots. (Both linoleic and linolenic acids are unsaturated fats that vary slightly in chemical structure. Your body needs both of them to work well.)

Clearly, reducing your intake of saturated fat and increasing your consumption of good fats will help to keep you heart working at its best. In addition, increasing your intake of antioxidants is another way to stay heart-healthy.

In recent years, much attention has been paid to antioxidants and their role in the prevention of heart disease. As you know, antioxidants protect against damage inflicted by free radicals, highly reactive atoms that in the body rapidly transfer their excess energy to another atom. In the process, free radicals give off heat, which can destroy healthy tissue.

Cholesterol is particularly vulnerable to free-radical attack, and in the process, it becomes oxidized. Once cholesterol is oxidized, it draws other cells to it, precipitating a snowball reaction that culminates in artery-clogging plaque. The more cholesterol around, the more damage is done.

As stated earlier, antioxidants are substances that prevent cells from being damaged by free radicals. The body produces many different types of antioxidants, including *superoxide dismutase,* an enzyme found within the cells, and gluthathione, an amino acid. Fruits and vegetables are also an excellent source of antioxidant vitamins and minerals, and they are also widely available in supplement form.

Antioxidants

Bioflavonoids—Bioflavonoids, a group of about five-hundred compounds, provide color to citrus fruits and vegetables. Some bioflavonoids are potent antioxidants that are believed to work in conjunction with vitamin C to improve the strength of small blood vessels or capillaries. Thus, bioflavonoids and other antioxidants found in produce and other foods may help protect against heart disease, because they appear to keep cholesterol in the blood from undergoing oxidation. Bioflavonoids may also help keep blood from becoming too thick and therefore more likely to clot. Researchers in Holland evaluated the diets of 805 men aged sixty-five to eighty-four. The group who consumed the highest amounts of bioflavonoids had the lowest rate of heart disease. Researchers speculated that the antioxidant action of bioflavonoids may prevent the oxidizing of LDL, or "bad" cholesterol.

Betacarotene—This superstar of the carotenoid family is found in food (raw carrots, cantaloupe, butternut squash, pumpkins, spinach, sweet potatoes, and broccoli) and may be effective in preventing or slowing the progression of atherosclerosis. Betacarotene, which is converted into vitamin A as the body needs it, is a potent antioxidant. Test-tube studies have shown that betacarotene can protect LDL cholesterol from oxidative damage caused by free radicals, which suggests that it will work the same way within the human body.

Vitamin C —Provocative new findings suggest that getting plenty of vitamin C provides greater protection against heart disease than either maintaining low blood cholesterol or eating a low-fat diet.

A study at the University of California at Los Angeles revealed a much lower death rate among those who took vitamin C supplements compared to people who had adequate vitamin C in their diets, but took no supplements. Researchers looked at the vitamin C intakes and death rates of more than eleven thousand men and women. As a group, the more vitamin C the men consumed, the fewer deaths they suffered from heart disease. For women the results were similar but less conclusive. The connection to prevention of heart disease to vitamin C has been linked to a reduced risk of high blood pressure and hardening of the arteries.

Another recent study at the University of California at Berkeley revealed that men who consumed very low levels of vitamin C (less than 20 milligrams) had a 50 percent drop in blood levels of glutathione, a compound that helps guard against heart disease. When the vitamin was restored, glutathione levels bounced back. Other studies have shown that vitamin C is particularly effective in intercepting oxidants before they can attack blood lipids. Fruits and vegetables, particularly green and citrus fruits, currants, strawberries, potatoes, turnips, and green leafy vegetables, provide important combinations of beneficial antioxidants and natural protective factors, including vitamin C. However, since few people get enough vitamin C from food, daily supplements of calcium ascorbate are recommended.

Vitamin E—Vitamin E is found in olive oil, a staple of Mediterranean countries, green leafy vegetables, soybeans, alfalfa, and sunflower and sesame seed. It is also available in supplement form. Many researchers believe that vitamin E might help prevent oxidation of LDL—the so-called "bad" cholesterol—and therefore may lower the risk of coronary heart disease in both men and women.

In one small study reported in *Circulation* (December 1993), researchers gave a group of men 800 IU of vitamin E. They found the vitamin protected LDL from the type of oxidative damage that can cause plaque and clog arteries.

If these results are confirmed in future studies, vitamin E may turn out to be the new star of the antioxidant mix in protecting both LDL and your blood vessels.

The Journal of Thoracic and Cardiovascular Surgery, (August 1994) reports that patients undergoing heart surgery (heart bypass and angioplasty procedures) who where given 447 IU of vitamin E for two weeks before surgery showed small improvements in chemical factors that indicated less damage to the heart muscle and returned to normal metabolic functions more quickly. No wonder that many cardiologists are now routinely prescribing Vitamin E supplements for their patients.

Selenium—Selenium, a mineral found in grains and seafood, may help to activate one of the most potent antioxidants, *glutathione peroxidase*. This antioxidant discourages free radicals from attacking LDL (bad) cholesterol.

In a recent study of 2,600 people reported in the *American Journal of Epidemiology* (June 1995), researchers found that those with higher blood selenium levels had a 60 percent lower risk of heart disease than people who had lower levels of this important mineral. Similar to other minerals such as fluoride, the levels of selenium in soil varies from region to region. Several studies have documented that people who live in areas where there is a high level of selenium in the soil (which presumably seeps into the food and water supply) have significantly lower levels of stroke that those who live in areas with low levels of selenium in the soil. In fact, because of the high rate of stroke and low levels of selenium in the soil, the selenium poor regions of the southwest United States have been dubbed the "stroke belt."

Niacin (Vitamin B3)—Niacin works with two other B vitamins, thiamin and riboflavin, in the metabolism of carbohydrates, and in recent years has gained fame as a potent cholesterol-lowering agent. In 1975, the Coronary Drug Project, a major study, reported that niacin could dramatically reduce cholesterol levels and, even better, reduced the rate of second heart attacks by 30 percent. A fifteen-year follow-up study comparing niacin to clofibrate, a cholesterol-lowering drug, found that even though both agents lowered cholesterol, patients who had taken the niacin had significantly fewer heart-related deaths than those who had taken the clofibrate.

High levels of niacin can produce unpleasant and sometimes dangerous side effects, including hot flushes and serious liver damage. If taken with chromium, niacin can be effective in lower doses. (If you take niacin, you should do so only under the supervision of your physician or natural healer.)

Folic acid—Recent studies show that folic acid, a B vitamin often called *folacin* or *folate*, may be an essential factor in warding off heart attacks and strokes, and that a less than optimal intake can double or triple the risk of developing heart disease.

A study of fifteen thousand male physicians by researchers in Massachusetts and Oregon revealed that the risk of suffering a heart attack was three times higher in those who had a high level of an amino acid called *homocysteine*.

Folate is involved in breaking down homocysteine, and when intake of the vitamin is low, homocysteine tends to build up in the blood. Researchers from the Framingham, Massachusetts, Heart Study and Tufts University in Boston have linked B-vitamin deficiency and cardiovascular disease. Elderly people with higher than normal levels of an amino acid called *homocysteine* had significant blockages in their carotid arteries (the arteries in the neck that deliver blood to the brain.) Of the 418 men and 623 women who took part in the study, those with the highest homocysteine levels had double the risk of having artery blockage. University of Washington researchers combined the results of thirty-eight studies of homocysteine, and reported in the *Journal of the American Medical Association* (Oct. 4, 1995) that 10 percent of the nation's heart disease was a result of high homocysteine levels.

Folic acid is found in navy beans, broccoli, orange juice, green leafy vegetables, fruits, and legumes, and in supplements.

Chromium—New research indicates that chromium may give good cholesterol a boost. In a new study, seventy-six heart-disease patients were treated daily with either chromium or a placebo for seven to sixteen months. They received 1250 micrograms daily (roughly five times the recommended amount). Those who took chromium had a dramatic jump in "good" HDL cholesterol, which represents a potential 30 percent reduction in heart disease risk. Chromium can be found in broccoli, turkey, ham, and grape juice.

Other Supplements

Coenzyme Q10—Coenzyme Q10 is found in every cell in the body. It is a nonprotein organic compound that, in the presence of an enzyme (a protein found in cells), plays an essential role in the chemical reaction that provides cells with energy. The potential therapeutic use of CoQ10 in cardiovascular disease has been clearly documented in both animal and human trials. In fact, heart-muscle biopsies in patients with various cardiac diseases showed a CoQ10 deficiency in 50 to 75 percent of cases.

CoQ10 has shown great promise in the treatment of heart disease including angina pectoris, congestive heart failure, mitral valve prolapse, and hypertension. Coenzyme Q10 is available in capsules.

L-carnitine—L-carnitine is a nonprotein amino acid that is found in heart and skeletal muscle. Its primary job is to carry fatty acids across the *mitochondria*—the so-called powerhouse of the cell—providing heart and skeletal cells with energy.

Several clinical trials have demonstrated that supplements of L-carnitine allow the heart to utilize its limited oxygen supply—thereby improving angina and ischemic heart disease (that is, when the heart is deprived of oxygen).

Red meat and dairy products are the best natural sources of L-carnitine but, unfortunately, these foods are also high in saturated fat. Therefore, an L-carnitine supplement might be the answer to keeping the diet low in fat while getting this helpful amino acid.

Soy protein—Researchers from the University of Kentucky in Lexington report that eating soy protein significantly reduces moderate-to-high concentrations of blood cholesterol. James T. Anderson, who led the study, pooled the results of thirty-eight clinical trials that included 730 men, women, and children and analyzed the effect of eating an average 57 grams of soy protein a day. As reported in *The New England Journal of Medicine,* volunteers who got half their protein from soy had their cholesterol concentrations drop an average of 10 percent.

Herbs

Green tea—At the National Institutes of Health, as well as at research centers throughout the United States and abroad, scientists are finding in preliminary studies that tea may help keep cholesterol from clogging arteries. Thus far, green tea, the type typically drunk in Asia, has received the bulk of scientific attention for the simple reason that most of this research has been done in Asia. Black tea, which is more commonly consumed in the West, has a slightly different chemical makeup, but so far lab tests indicate it may also have the same preventive properties as green tea.

Garlic—Research indicates that garlic may play a significant role in the prevention of the oxidation of LDL, and may actually prevent the liver from producing excess fat and cholesterol. In a study at the Clinical Research Center and Tulane University School of Medicine, New Orleans, forty-two healthy adults received either 300 mg. three times daily of standardized garlic powder in tablet form or a placebo. The result showed a significant reduction in serum total cholesterol and in LDL cholesterol in those taking the garlic supplement. In test-tube studies, Japanese researchers have documented the antioxidant- and free-radical—scavenging effects of aged garlic extract.

Hawthorn—Since the late 19th century, hawthorn has been used successfully for various heart diseases, including geriatric or stressed heart, hypertension, coronary insufficiency, heart attack, damage to coronary arteries, and angina pectoris. Hawthorn extracts have been shown to dilate coronary blood vessels, thus improving the flow of blood to the heart. At the same time, this herb helps strengthen the heart muscle and works to help the body rid itself of excess salt and water.

Tumeric—If you eat curry, you have tasted this exotic spice that adds flavor and color to many foods, including curry powder and sauces. Studies show that tumeric can lower blood-cholesterol levels by stimulating the production of bile. Bile is produced by the liver, and cholesterol is a component of bile—thus when the production of bile increases, it uses excess cholesterol. Tumeric also prevents the formation of dangerous blood clots that can lead to heart attack.

Ginkgo biloba—This ancient herb can help improve the flow of blood throughout the body. It is also an antioxidant, which means that it slows the formation of compounds called free radicals, those nasty molecules that are responsible for the oxidation of cholesterol.

Alfalfa—The leaves of the alfalfa plant help reduce blood-cholesterol levels and plaque deposits on artery walls. Alfalfa sprouts have a similar effect.

Ginger—This root is another cholesterol buster and also helps lower blood pressure and prevents blood clots.

Personal Advice

First things first. If you smoke, quit. Despite what tobacco executives would lead you to believe, the evidence linking smoking to heart disease is overwhelming. Cigarette smoke is full of chemicals that can inflict great harm to your heart and to the rest of your body.

If you're overweight, lose weight. While no one can argue that exercise reduces the risk of coronary-artery disease, a new study at the University of Maryland School of Medicine concluded that exercise without weight loss will not significantly improve coronary-artery disease risk factors in overweight, middle-aged and older men. The researchers concluded that losing weight is an essential first step toward achieving cardiovascular health.

However, the report suggests that weight loss without exercise won't work, because without an increase in physical activity, maintaining weight loss is unlikely and simply begins a vicious cycle of losing and regaining unwanted pounds.

The best way to lose weight is to eat less and exercise more. A regular program of aerobic exercise can raise the metabolic rate and thus increase the number of calories used, both during the activity and between exercise sessions. Exercise also helps to relieve emotional stresses that prompt many people to overeat.

If you are stressed out, learn how to relax (if you want to know how, see page 42). Unrelenting stress can have a toxic effect on the body and contribute to coronary disease by raising blood pressure and inflicting injury to the heart muscle itself. In addition, stressful situations like driving in heavy traffic or racing to beat a deadline at work, and living with unrelieved anger and hostility can cause an increase in heart rate which, in turn, can lead to a dangerous arrhythmia.

Earl's Rx

These supplements will keep you heart healthy.

Antioxidant multivitamin: Any of the numerous broad-spectrum antioxidant multivitamin formulas sold today will offer excellent protection against heart disease. A good antioxidant formula should include alpha and betacarotene, vitamin C, vitamin E, and selenium. Take one to two tablets or capsules daily, as directed.

L-carnitine: One or two 500 mg. capsules daily.

Garlic: One 500 mg. raw, aged odorless garlic daily.

Niacin and chromium piccolinate: Take one 500 mg. "no-flush" niacin with inositol hexanicotinate and 600 mcg. of chromium piccolinate daily. (Niacin can produce hot flushes in some people. Although this is harmless, it can be very uncomfortable.)

Folic acid: One 400 mcg. tablet daily.

Magnesium: One 500 mg. capsule or tablet daily.

Coenzyme Q10: One 100 mg. tablet or capsule up to three times daily.

Soy Protein: One to three ounces daily. (Soy shakes are available in powder form and can be mixed in water or juice, or it can be used in cooking.)

Green tea: Two tablets daily (or drink three cups of decaffeinated tea).

Ginkgo biloba: Three 60 mg. capsules or tablets daily.

Herpes

Between 20 and 40 percent of Americans have recurrent herpes infections.

Supplements can help reduce the recurrence of infection and lessen its duration.

H erpes is a virtual epidemic in the United States. It is one of the most common of all infections, and one of the most difficult to beat.

There are several types of herpes viruses; the ones that are most prevalent are *Herpes Simplex Type I* and *Herpes Simplex Type II.*

Herpes Simplex Type I is characterized by fever blisters on or around the mouth—what we often call *cold sores.* Herpes Simplex Type II causes genital herpes, or blisters in the genital area. Either form of herpes is painful, and can lie dormant for years before striking without notice.

Almost everyone is exposed to the herpes virus at some time in their lives, but not everyone develops clinical infection. To me, this clearly shows that the immune system acts as a defense mechanism in protecting against the herpes virus, and that enhancing the immune system can go a long way toward preventing herpes outbreaks of any type.

Vitamin and Mineral Combinations

Zinc and Vitamin C—Clinical studies suggest that zinc and vitamin C supplements taken orally reduce the symptoms of herpes simplex. In one study, doctors gave patients 250 mg. of vitamin C and 100 mg. of zinc twice daily for six weeks. Symptoms were relieved as long as the subjects continued to take the supplements.

Vitamin C may work against herpes because it increases the levels of *glutathione,* a protein building amino acid that is a powerful virus fighter. A recent study at Arizona State University showed that 500 mg. of vitamin C daily increases the body's production of glutathione by close to 50 percent.

The topical application of zinc-sulfate solutions have also been shown to be effective in both easing symptoms and inhibiting recurrences of herpes.

Amino Acids

Lysine—Doctors at the Indiana School of Medicine gave 800 to 1000 mg. of lysine daily to forty-five patients with active herpes infections. The supplements helped stop the pain of the herpes eruption overnight for most of the patients, and all but three had a complete disappearance of symptoms within a few days.

Lysine suppresses the amino acid *arginine*, which promotes viral growth. It might also help to minimize your intake of arginine-rich foods such as almonds and other nuts, chocolate, carob, and seeds, and increase your intake of lysine-rich foods such as most vegetables, legumes, fish, turkey, and chicken.

Herbs

Echinacea—The healing power of this herb was well-known to Native Americans, who introduced it to the settlers. Around the turn of the century, scientists who had studied echinacea observed that this herb could boost our ability to resist disease. Once antibiotics were discovered, scientists turned away from traditional remedies, but interest was renewed in the 1970s when it became apparent that antibiotics could cause as many problems as they cured. One of the most fascinating studies of echinacea was done in Germany in 1978. Researchers pretreated cells from both humans and animals with echinacea, and then infected them with influenza, herpes, and canker sore viruses.

The results showed that a four-to-six hour pretreatment with echinacea increased the cells' resistance to subsequent infection by 50 to 80 percent, and maintained that resistance for the next forty-eight hours. When you feel a herpes attack coming on, reach for the echinacea!

Mint—This member of the *melissa officinalis* family is included in many different commercial creams for herpes that are sold primarily in natural-food stores. When the cream was applied to the skin eruption caused by the herpes-simplex virus in test patients, it interrupted the infection quickly and promoted faster healing of the herpes blisters.

Balm—Another member of the *melissa officinalis* family, balm has been used for thousands of years in Ancient Greece, the Middle East, and Asia, to treat a variety of illnesses, including skin wounds. Skin creams containing balm are very effective in treating cold sores caused by the herpes-simplex virus.

Garlic—No wonder studies have shown that garlic can be effective against chronic herpes infection—it is a proven immune enhancer.

Siberian ginseng—This traditional Chinese herb is well-known for its ability to stimulate the immune system. If you are battling chronic herpes infection, Siberian ginseng may give your immune system the added boost it needs to fight the infection.

Tea tree oil—A solution made from tea tree oil has also been shown effective in lessening the pain and duration of cold sores caused by the herpes-simplex virus when applied directly to the infected area.

Personal Advice

Prevention can go a long way in helping to control herpes. It's just common sense to avoid sexual contact with someone who has an active case of herpes. Using a condom can also help to prevent the spread of herpes virus.

If you have a history of herpes, avoid getting overtired or allowing yourself to get run down. When you are fatigued, your immune system cannot function as well, and you may be more vulnerable to a recurrence of herpes.

Earl's Rx

If you are prone to herpes infection, I recommend the following immune-strengthening regimen.

Echinacea: Take 500 mg. capsules, one to three times daily.

Lysine: Take 1000 mg. capsules, three to four times daily, on an empty stomach.

Zinc: One 50 mg. tablet or capsule daily.

Vitamin C: Two 500 mg. capsules or tablets daily of calcium ascorbate, taken with food.

To relieve the discomfort of cold sores, apply tea tree oil directly to the abrasion several times daily.

Salves containing a combination of mint, balm, and/or tea tree oil are available in natural food stores, and are not only very soothing, but can promote healing. Gently apply the salve directly to the cold sore several times daily.

High Blood Pressure

About 63 million Americans have high blood pressure.

High blood pressure typically strikes after the age of thirty and is slightly more common in women than in men after the age of fifty.

It is called the *silent killer* because it rarely causes symptoms until complications occur.

Compared to whites, African Americans have a much higher risk of high blood pressure.

High blood pressure is the most common of all of the cardiovascular diseases and, in my opinion, one of the most preventable. Simply by controlling factors such as weight, diet, and stress, you can dramatically reduce your risk of developing this common and potentially lethal problem. In addition, there are several supplements that are proven winners in the war against high blood pressure.

High blood pressure is a particularly insidious disease because there are few symptoms in its early stages, and many people who have high blood pressure are completely unaware of it. In the case of high blood pressure, ignorance is not bliss. If left untreated, this initially benign disease can lead to heart attack, stroke, kidney failure, and atherosclerosis.

Blood pressure is the pressure, or tension, of the blood within the arteries of the circulatory system. When the heart pumps, it causes the blood to flow through the large arteries into the smaller arteries. In order to keep the blood flowing throughout the body, the arteries must contract and expand. Contraction of the small arteries increases the resistance to blood flow, while expansion has the opposite effect. The contraction and expansion regulates the rate of flow of blood from the heart throughout the circulatory system. When the inside of the arteries remain constricted, they can create a condition of *hypertension,* or high blood pressure.

Arterial blood pressure is written as *systolic* pressure over *diastolic* pressure. Systolic pressure is the maximum blood pressure that occurs during the contraction of the heart; diastolic pressure is the minimum pressure measured during the resting period of the heart.

Much controversy exists about what constitutes normal and elevated blood pressure levels. Scientists have determined that there is no ideal pressure for everyone. Instead, they have determined that acceptable blood pressure falls within a range rather than being a particular pair of numbers.

The official definition of high blood pressure is a reading of more than 140/90. In recent years, however, many physicians have come to believe that this is too high, and that even a diastolic (bottom number) reading of more than 80 should be viewed as too high.

What's so bad about high blood pressure? When blood pressure is high, the heart has to work harder than normal to pump enough blood and oxygen to the body's organs and tissues which puts both the heart and the arteries under great strain. This in turn can cause the heart to enlarge and the arteries to become scarred, hardened, narrowed, and less elastic. If the body's organs don't get enough oxygen and nutrients, they can't function properly, and there's also the risk that a blood clot may lodge in a narrowed artery, which can cause a heart attack or stroke.

Hypertension may be one of the most common of all medical problems, but its cause is still very much a mystery. In fact, in more than 90 percent of patients with hypertension, an underlying cause cannot be positively identified. This is called *primary hypertension*. We do know that factors such as diet, stress, and obesity can affect blood pressure in otherwise healthy people. A small number of people have secondary hypertension, which is due to a specific problem. Some of the causes of secondary hypertension include diseases of the kidney or adrenal gland, narrowing of the artery that supplies the kidney, congenital narrowing of the aorta, and the use of birth control pills.

Diet appears to play a role in the regulation of blood pressure. In some people, excessive salt intake can raise blood pressure, because to keep the body functioning properly, a normal salt-to-water ratio must be achieved. The more salt you take in, the more water you retain, which will increase the amount of fluid circulating throughout the body. The added fluid load places an additional strain on the arteries and the heart, and can increase blood pressure. Very often, simply cutting back on salt can help to reduce blood pressure.

There are numerous prescription drugs that are used to control high blood pressure, including diuretics, which reduce the fluid load. Nearly all work well but nearly all have some side effects from fatigue to depression to impotence. For most people, a combination of diet and natural supplements can eliminate or greatly reduce the need for drugs.

Minerals

Calcium—Calcium is best known as the mineral that helps to keep teeth and bones strong, but it soon may also gain fame as the mineral that can lower blood pressure. More than eighty studies have shown that calcium supplements help *lower* blood pressure in some people with high blood pressure. However, a new study suggests calcium may also help *prevent* high blood pressure.

Researchers at the University of Southern California School of Medicine in Los Angeles studied more than 6,600 men and women for a period of thirteen years. None of the participants suffered from high blood pressure at the study's start, but many of the volunteers did develop high blood pressure during the study. Calcium consumption, based on dietary questions, was measured. The researchers discovered that people who consumed at least 1 gram of calcium per day (1000 mg.) lowered their risk of high blood pressure by about 12 percent.

What is even more exciting is the fact that those under age forty who consumed 1000 mg. of calcium daily reduced their risk of high blood pressure by 25 percent. Among people under forty who were normal weight and moderate drinkers, the decrease was even greater: These people reduced their risk of high blood pressure by nearly 40 percent. (Although moderate alcohol consumption has beneficial effects on blood pressure, more than two drinks daily can actually raise blood pressure.) This study suggests that if taken early enough in life, calcium, along with other sensible health habits, may be a potent force against high blood pressure. This new study also confirms previous research showing that calcium supplements prevent *preeclampsia,* a type of high blood pressure that can develop during pregnancy.

Potassium—Potassium is a powerful protector against high blood pressure. This mineral is a member of a group of nutrients called *electrolytes,* which regulate the balance of fluid in the body, regulate the heartbeat, and also control the electrical impulses created by nerve and muscle cells. There are several ways that potassium might benefit blood-pressure regulation. First, potassium is a natural diuretic. Diuretics reduce the amount of fluid in the body and, since there is less fluid to pump through the heart, it reduces the workload on the heart and blood vessels which, in turn, lowers blood pressure. Second, potassium inhibits specific enzymes and hormones that cause blood pressure to rise. Third, potassium relaxes the muscles that line the blood-vessel walls, thus causing less resistance to blood flow and reduced blood pressure.

Ideally, potassium intake should be greater than sodium intake and, considering that people in North America may consume as much as 18,000 mg. of sodium daily and as little as 1,500 mg. of potassium, it is easy to see that the great amount of sodium compared to potassium could have an adverse effect on blood pressure.

As I noted earlier, African Americans are at particular risk of developing high blood pressure. To make matters worse, for reasons that are not fully understood, African Americans are often less responsive to conventional drug therapies and more likely to develop complications from high blood pressure, such as kidney disorders and stroke. A recent study, however, suggests that potassium may work well in lowering blood pressure for African Americans. A study reported by F.L. Brancati, M.D., at the American Heart Association's 67th Scientific Sessions in Dallas, showed reduced blood pressure in forty-three African Americans who took potassium supplements for three weeks. In contrast, average blood pressure in forty-four healthy African Americans who received a placebo did not change. Given the fact that potassium is safe and inexpensive, I think it makes sense for everyone with even borderline high blood pressure to take potassium supplements, but it is of special importance for African Americans.

Potassium may also help people who are already taking drugs for hypertension. A study at the University of Naples, Italy, concluded that increasing the dietary potassium intake from natural foods is an effective way to reduce the need for medication to lower blood pressure. Foods that are high in potassium include bananas, dried apricots, potatoes, orange juice, potatoes, cauliflower, squash, and plain low-fat yogurt.

Magnesium—In a recent Dutch study, ninety-one middle-aged and elderly women with mild high blood pressure were treated with no other medication than magnesium. The results: Six months of magnesium supplements reduced the systolic pressure by an average of 2.7 percent and the diastolic pressure by an average of 3.4 percent. Dietary sources of magnesium include beans, brown rice and other grains, popcorn, nuts, spinach, broccoli, green peas, corn, acorn squash, white and sweet potatoes, fish, and skim milk.

Other Supplements

Omega-3 fatty acids—New research suggests that omega-3 fatty acids found in fatty fish may have a positive effect on the walls of blood vessels, which may help to normalize blood pressure.

L-carnitine—L-carnitine is a nonprotein acid that is found in heart and skeletal muscle. L-carnitine allows the heart to utilize a limited oxygen supply, thus improving angina and ischemic heart disease, which is caused by a reduction in blood flow to the heart. L-carnitine has been shown to reduce blood pressure in heart patients, and from this we can assume that it would have an equally beneficial effect on healthy people.

Herbs

Hawthorn—The use of hawthorn for heart conditions dates back to the seventeenth century. Since the late nineteenth century, hawthorn has been used successfully for various heart diseases, including angina pectoris (chest pain), arrhythmia, and as a heart tonic to regulate circulation. Studies on humans and animals have shown that this herb can lower blood pressure during exertion, as well as strengthen the heart's ability to pump blood. Hawthorn is a natural diuretic that helps the body rid itself of excess salt and water.

Natural diuretics—Other natural herbal diuretics include astragalus, buchu, burdock, horehound, juniper berries, uva ursi (also known as bearberry,) wild Oregon grape, and dong quai.

Foods that aid in helping the body get rid of excess water include celery, alfalfa, artichoke, asparagus, cucumber, dandelion, and sarsaparilla.

Personal Advice

Eat well, exercise, relax, stop smoking, and drink alcohol moderately, if at all, and you will greatly reduce the risk of high blood pressure.

Lose weight—If you are overweight, there is no more effective way to reduce your blood pressure than to shed those excess pounds. I have literally seen blood pressure levels plummet as the pounds roll off. Clinical studies have also repeatedly demonstrated that obesity is a major factor in hypertension, so weight control should be high on the list of preventatives.

Sugar and salt intake should be restricted, while foods rich in potassium, magnesium, and fiber should be encouraged. Salt shows up in a great many food products like bread, canned foods, and processed foods, so label reading should become a habit. In addition, a low-total-fat diet (with moderate levels of linoleic acid found in fatty fish, safflower oil, and soybean oil) should help maintain cardiovascular health. Garlic and other members of the onion family should be freely consumed—they add flavor without salt.

Although effects of long-term caffeine consumption on blood pressure have not yet been unequivocally determined, short-term studies show elevations in blood pressure in adults who drank five or more cups of coffee a day compared to noncoffee drinkers.

Relax and live longer!—Stress reduction is a major risk reducer for all heart-related disease. Relaxation techniques such as biofeedback, meditation, yoga, progressive muscle relaxation, and exercise are all proven ways to help reduce stress.

Earl's Rx

Calcium: Take 1000 mg. of calcium citrate daily with 400 IU of vitamin D.

Magnesium: One (500 mg.) capsule or tablet daily.

Potassium: Take three 99 mg. tablets daily (plus eat 1–2 bananas daily).

Fish oil capsules: Three to six 1000 mg. capsules daily.

L-carnitine: Two 500 mg. capsules or tablets daily, taken between meals.

Hypoglycemia

Only 1 percent of the population has true hypoglycemia, but many other people experience related symptoms.

Diet and supplements can help to prevent the sugar highs and lows.

About a decade ago, hypoglycemia was a fairly common diagnosis, in fact, it seemed that nearly everyone had, or thought they had, "low blood sugar." At that time, if a women, in particular, went to the doctor with unspecified or vague complaints (especially when the main one was exhaustion) she was very likely to come away with a diagnosis of hypoglycemia. (For some unexplained reason, this condition is diagnosed much more often in women than in men.) Today, that diagnosis is losing favor. That's not surprising because true hypoglycemia is rare and is usually connected to another disease, such as diabetes.

True hypoglycemia is an abnormally low concentration of glucose (sugar) in the blood. It is generally caused by the failure of certain body systems to replenish supplies of blood glucose as they are depleted. This causes symptoms that include fatigue, confusion, nervousness, sweating, insomnia, moodiness, dizziness—and in extreme cases—convulsions or coma. In the case of diabetics, they do not have enough insulin to properly utilize blood sugar. (See "Diabetes," p. 111.)

The good news is that true hypoglycemia affects less than 1 percent of healthy people, and an accurate diagnosis can be made by taking a simple blood-sugar test. Why, then, do so many people think they suffer from it, and why was it so frequently diagnosed? Although most people do not have bona fide hypoglycemia, they may experience many of the same symptoms, often due to diet. The problem can be caused by eating foods that cause sugar levels to drop either too low or too quickly. These foods include refined carbohydrates, candy, caffeine, and sugary desserts.

This is how it works: Soon after eating, the level of sugar in the blood starts to go up. As blood sugar rises, the pancreas responds by releasing the hormone insulin, which allows glucose to leave the bloodstream and enter our various tissues, where it fuels the body's activities. Some sugar is also stored in liver for later use. Then, when the body uses up the sugar, insulin levels drop, which keeps sugar in the blood at a steady level.

However, if we feel we need a pick-me-up we might be tempted to eat a candy bar, or indulge in a hot-fudge sundae. What happens then is that the pancreas overreacts and starts pumping out the insulin, sugar levels plunge, and a vicious cycle of fluctuation in sugar levels begins.

The confusion in diagnosis may actually be due to a failure to recognize different types of hypoglycemia. *Reactive hypoglycemia* is a low blood sugar condition caused by a reaction to food. This occurs when sugar levels fall low enough to cause the hormone adrenaline to work hard to release stored sugar from the liver. Since adrenaline is also the hormone released during emergencies, the symptoms of reactive hypoglycemia can include rapid heartbeat, sweating, and trembling.

Fasting hypoglycemia, occurs in response to fasting, usually after about eight hours or more. Symptoms tend to be more severe and can include fainting, memory loss, seizure, and confusion. Eating regular meals can help to relieve this problem for most people. In rare cases, fasting hypoglycemia can be the result of a serious disorder such as a tumor of the pancreas so, to be on the safe side, anyone with these symptoms should be checked by his or her doctor.

What makes diagnosing this condition even more difficult is the fact that some people can have both kinds of hypoglycemia—that is, they can be affected by what they eat and by how often they eat. A change in diet and the addition of a few supplements may be of great help in alleviating their symptoms.

Minerals

Chromium—This essential trace element helps the body to utilize insulin and thus stabilize blood-sugar levels. Researchers tested eight women who took 200 mcg. of chromium daily for three months. All had their hypoglycemic symptoms eased, that is, they no longer experienced those sugar highs and lows. In diabetics who have *hyperglycemia* (too much sugar in the blood), chromium can lower both blood-sugar levels and the need for insulin.

Magnesium—This mineral, which is essential for converting blood sugar into energy, may also help to maintain normal blood-sugar levels. One double-blind study showed that 57 percent of hypoglycemic subjects who took daily magnesium supplements felt better, compared to 25 percent of those who were given a placebo.

Glutathione—This combination of three amino acids, glutamate, glycine, and cysteine is a potent antioxidant that deactivates free radicals and has been used to help in the treatment of diabetes and hypoglycemia.

Personal Advice

If you fill up on a lot of sugar-laden foods, chances are you are not eating enough essential nutrients, including calcium and magnesium. Your diet may also be deficient in other essential vitamins and trace minerals, including the B vitamins, chromium, zinc, and essential amino acids. These nutrients participate in various body enzyme systems and serve as precursors in the manufacture of hormones and neurotransmitters.

What to do? If you feel tired, light-headed, or edgy because you've been too busy to eat, don't reach for a candy bar; try a protein snack instead. Better yet, don't let yourself get into that condition in the first place. Eat five to six small meals a day rather than three large ones. That will stabilize the release of glucose into the blood.

Meals should contain not just carbohydrate, but also protein and some fat. For instance, a mid-morning snack of a slice of turkey, a few crackers, and perhaps a small glass of milk would be better than a glass of orange juice, or a cherry Danish. Caffeine and alcohol seem to interfere with the liver's ability to release stored sugar, so it makes sense to eliminate or cut back on those two items. A general overall good diet should include portions of fresh fruits and vegetables; meat, fish, or fowl, and carbohydrates.

Earl's Rx

Chromium picolinate: One 200 mcg. tablet or capsule three times daily.

Magnesium: One 500 mg. capsule or tablet daily.

Glutathione: One 500 mg. capsule one half hour before meals up to twice daily.

Immune Weakness

A strong immune system is the key to good health.

B ack in the late 1970s, I remember reading a newspaper account of an international meeting of prominent immunologists in which these learned men and women unequivocally declared that thanks to the widespread availability of antibiotics and the growing use of immunization, we had won the war against infectious disease. In other words, there was no contagious disease on the face of the planet that we could not defeat.

In fact, some immunologists were so confident that they could cure even the most lethal of diseases, they wondered out loud if they should consider pursuing another line of research!

Today, their statements seem almost laughable. Since the 1970s, millions of people worldwide have become infected with AIDS, a disease caused by a particularly vicious virus that destroys the body's own ability to fight against infection. To date, there is no cure. Only recently have scientists found a treatment that has yielded good results in some patients in keeping the virus under control, at least in the short run. In addition, the recent outbreak of ebola virus in Kenya showed just how quickly a persistent, highly contagious and deadly virus could do its dirty work. And it's not just viruses that are out of control. Doctors are fighting an equally uphill battle against antibiotic-resistant bacteria that are producing new and more lethal forms of tuberculosis, strep, and other ailments that we once thought could be easily controlled by drugs.

The same researchers who believed that they could control disease from the outside in by administering drugs and other therapies are now beginning to see that the way to eradicate disease is from the inside out, that is, by strengthening the body's own defense, the immune system. In recent years, we have learned a great deal about this remarkable mechanism that preserves our health and, from this knowledge, we have learned ways to enhance and protect it.

The *immune system* is a highly sophisticated network of specialized cells that defends the body against foreign organisms such as bacteria, viruses, and parasites, and guards against the growth of cancers.

The immune system works by stimulating the production of antibodies and cells which destroy or neutralize foreign bodies.

But as we age, the system becomes forgetful, that is, some of the body's immune cells that are programmed to distinguish friend from foe die off. Consequently, the system no longer remembers the good guys from the bad, and viruses and bacteria are allowed to flourish and something as simple as a cold or sore throat, which is easily defeated when we are young, is allowed to flourish and become dangerous as we age.

What is equally problematic is that when the immune system becomes so forgetful it attacks the body's own tissues and organs, causing catastrophic ailments. That is why autoimmune disorders such as rheumatoid arthritis are more common among the elderly.

The question is: How do you keep your immune system in peak condition? We do not have all the answers yet, but there is good evidence that many supplements can help to maintain strong, youthful immune function.

Minerals

Zinc—Zinc is a major player in the immune system, and studies have shown that many older people are deficient in this mineral. This may be because the elderly do not get enough zinc in their diets, and/or because their bodies are not absorbing zinc effectively.

Researchers at Wayne State University in Detroit gave zinc supplements (30 mg. a day) to thirteen zinc-deficient elderly men and women. After six months of extra zinc, they found significant improvements in several signs of immune function, including increased blood levels of a substance called *thymulin*. Without enough thymulin, of which zinc is a key ingredient, we can't make the mature T cells that are the body's front line of defense against foreign invaders.

Good zinc sources are meat, poultry, oysters, green peas, lentils, and fortified cereals, and it is also available in supplement form.

Selenium—Selenium, another antioxidant, is another immune booster. In one study, mice on selenium-deprived diets succumbed to an ordinarily harmless virus that they should have been able to easily defeat. Selenium is an antioxidant and, in all probability, works by helping to protect the immune system by damage from free radicals.

Vitamins

Betacarotene—Unless you have been living on another planet, you know by now that ultraviolet-A light from the sun can cause the skin to age, wrinkle, and become cancerous. What you may not have known is that ultraviolet light can inflict serious damage *inside* the body as well, especially to the immune system. Several studies have documented that ultraviolet-A light can lessen the ability of the immune system to wage an effective attack against foreign invaders and can leave us defenseless against cancer cells.

Scientists are testing the possibility that betacarotene may protect against ultraviolet-A's negative effect on immune function. In one study, researchers at Cornell University and Hoffman-LaRoche, Inc., divided twenty-four men into two groups. One group were given 30 mg. supplements of betacarotene, and the other group got a placebo. Then all twenty-four men were exposed to UVA light twelve times over two weeks, followed by blood tests to measure immune reaction to various types of antigens.

The men with low blood levels of betacarotene showed a weakened immune response to antigens. The men in the supplement group had immune systems that remained strong. Another reason to use that sunscreen—and another reason to eat plenty of yellow, orange, or green leafy vegetables, and shellfish.

Since betacarotene may give the immune system a boost, there is an intriguing possibility it can help prevent people who are infected with HIV from developing full blown AIDS. When twenty-one HIV-positive people were given 180 mg. (3000,00 IU) of betacarotene every day for four weeks, their disease-fighting T-cell activity increased significantly. Those who were given placebos had a continual drop in T-cell activity. More testing is necessary on a larger scale to confirm these results, but eating betacarotene-rich foods certainly can't hurt!

Vitamin E—Of all the nutrients linked to the healthy functioning of the immune system, vitamin E shows the most promise. Researchers supplemented the diets of healthy adults with 800 IUs of vitamin E daily for thirty days, followed by testing of immune-system response. All showed significant increases in immune response.

Vitamin E may suppress the production of *prostaglandins*, hormone-like compounds that can cause inflammation and have been linked to age-related declines in immune function. Other research suggests that E enhances the performance of the T-cells that help fight viral and bacterial infection, by protecting them against damage from free radicals.

Good sources of Vitamin E are grains, seeds, nuts, wheat germ, and dark leafy greens like spinach and kale; it is also available in supplements.

Vitamin B6—Several studies have revealed a link between low levels of B6 and poor immune response in both humans and animals. Animal studies have shown that B6 deficiency will adversely affect the function of the *thymus*, a small gland located at the breast bone in which the all-important T cells are stored. If the thymus is not functioning normally, it can impair the ability of T cells to fight infection. Several studies have also shown that B6 deficiency will lead to impaired antibody production, which means that the immune system will not be able to produce the foot soldiers—the disease-fighting cells—needed to carry out its orders. Vitamin B6 also plays a critical role in the metabolism of nucleic acids and in protein synthesis, both of which are essential for the immune system to function well. Therefore, a deficiency of this nutrient could have a profound effect on your ability to produce a normal immune response.

Vitamin C—Vitamin C can protect against viral infection. (See "Colds," p. 96.)

Herbs and Fruits

Aloe—More than 6,000 years ago Egyptians were using aloe to treat disease and, if animal studies hold true for humans, aloe shows promise as a potent immune-enhancing drug. Researchers at the College of Veterinary Medicine at Texas A&M University have recently shown that the plant has a remarkable effect on tumors in mice and horses. Aloe works by stimulating the release of natural substances in the body that turn on the immune system. To date, it is only approved for veterinary uses, but human clinical trials are being conducted in Canada on patients with AIDS, and trials for other applications are expected.

Garlic—From Ancient Greece and Rome, from Asia to the Middle East, for thousands of years garlic has been in the forefront of antibacterial treatment. With the discovery of antibiotics, garlic began to take a back seat. Now with the appearance of supergerms that resist antibiotics, garlic is back on the list of infection fighters. It is available in capsules, powder, and oil, and, of course, in its natural form.

What I like best about natural herbs like garlic is they do not attack bacteria indiscriminately or suppress the body's natural immune defenses the way antibiotic drugs do. They are probiotic, stimulating the body's natural defense mechanisms, without harming "friendly" bacteria.

Echinacea—Echinacea was well known to Native Americans of the Great Plains who used it as a general cure-all, especially for infections. At one time it was one of the most prescribed medicines in the United States. In the early 1900s, echinacea was used by doctors to treat just about everything from boils to poison ivy to appendicitis. After the antibiotic revolution, interest in echinacea waned, but this herb has been recently rediscovered by a new generation who now recognize that the so-called wonder drugs are not so wonderful, and that the best way to fight disease is by fortifying our own defenses naturally.

Europeans, especially German researchers, have studied echinacea extensively, and there are hundreds of research papers that can attest to its immune-enhancing properties.

Astragalus—This herb has long been utilized in Chinese medicine. Recent studies have shown that astragalus may induce interferon production (our disease-fighting cells) kill viruses, and destroy cancer cells.

Goldenseal—This Native American plant was widely used by healers for sore eyes and skin diseases. Recent research has corroborated its antibacterial properties. (Goldenseal should not be used for more than two weeks at a time since, overexposure will lessen its effect on the body. This herb should not be used during pregnancy.)

Barberry—This fruit contains *berberine,* a remarkable infection fighter that may stimulate the immune system. Studies show that it activates the *macrophages,* white blood cells that circulate throughout the bloodstream devouring harmful microorganisms.

Oregon grape—This fruit is a close cousin of barberry and is also believed to be an immune stimulant.

Osha—The root of this plant stimulates resistance to viral infections and may help reduce the discomfort and inflammation associated with respiratory infections.

Other Supplements

Glutathione—This peptide, which contains three amino acids—glutamic acid, cysteine, and glycine—functions as a coenzyme in reducing oxidative damage. Studies indicate glutathione supplements can give an ailing immune system a much-needed boost, especially in older people.

Melatonin—Melatonin, a hormone produced in the pineal gland (a tiny gland in the brain) has recently been touted for its ability to slow down the aging process, but it also appears to be a potent immune enhancer. One of the major benefits of melatonin is that it may help to prevent the loss of immune-cell memory.

Researchers have found that when melatonin was added to the nighttime drinking water of older mice, it had some dramatic effects. First, it increased the weight of the *thymus,* a small gland found at the base of the neck in which immune cells are produced, and helped restore the "memory" of the T cells, important disease-fighting cells. Thus, in test-tube studies, the cells were able to remember potential threats and to eliminate them.

Another study investigated how a loss of melatonin would affect the body's ability to manufacture antibodies. Mice were given drugs to reduce the effectiveness of the pineal gland, which produces melatonin, and an immediate drop in antibody production was noted. When the melatonin was added to their drinking water, their immune system bounced back.

Stress can have a devastating effect on the immune system. Studies show that mice who were subjected to extreme stress suffered a loss in immune response. When given melatonin supplements, their immune response rebounded and they were able to counteract some of the most debilitating health effects of stress.

After death and taxes, one thing is inevitable: Whenever we go for long periods of time without enough sleep, we get sick. According to researchers, sleep deprivation causes a sharp decline in immune function. Melatonin works to regulate the body's internal time-clocks, which regulate sleep patterns, helping the body to restore its immune function. (See "Sleep Disorders," p. 242.)

DHEA—DHEA is a hormone produced by the adrenal glands, the skin and the brain; as we age, our levels of DHEA decline. Many researchers believe that the lower levels of DHEA (and other key hormones) may be one reason our immune systems do not function as well as we get older. Dr. Omid Khorram, formerly a professor of medicine at the University of California at San Diego and now a member of the University of Wisconsin faculty, undertook a groundbreaking human study of DHEA and immune function. His is a particularly significant scientific investigation, because it is the longest study of the effect of restoring DHEA to youthful levels in otherwise healthy, older people. In Dr. Khoramm's study, nine healthy older men took DHEA for five months. Dr. Khorram found that DHEA did indeed have a palpable, measurable, rejuvenating effect on their aging immune systems. He found that DHEA elevated the men's levels of IGF-1, which is another potent immune enhancer produced by the body. DHEA stimulated the production of B cells, which produce the antibodies that fight viruses and bacteria, as well as the production of macrophages, the white blood cells that fight infection by "chewing up" infecting organisms. It increased the number and activity of cancer-fighting NK (natural killer) cells, which keep a watchful eye on potential cancerous cells and destroy them before they can grow. Dr. Khorram found that DHEA clearly restored a more youthful response pattern to the immune system of his human subjects.

Interestingly, Dr. Khorram hypothesizes that DHEA may work its magic on the immune system by virtue of an indirect path. He believes that DHEA controls the effect of stress-steroid hormones which, as I discussed earlier earlier, have a dampening effect effect on the immune system. By neutralizing these enemies of the immune system, DHEA indirectly bolsters it function.

Personal Advice

All supplements work best as part of a healthy lifestyle. Don't forget the importance of a good diet. Recently, researchers begun to confirm the relationship between nutritional status and immune function among the elderly who exhibit an increased incidence of *immune senescence* (impaired physical and mental ability). Studies confirmed that adequate intake of protein and calories can reverse this process and improve immune function in some cases.

Watch the sugar!—Sugar consumption—especially of refined white sugar—dramatically inhibits immune function by reducing the ability of neutrophils to engulf and destroy bacteria. (Neutrophils are white blood cells primarily responsible for defense against bacteria.) Alcohol has been shown to increase susceptibility to infections, probably by also depressing the level of neutrophils.

Other causes of immune suppression include food allergies, reactions to additives and chemicals in foods, and prolonged exposure to dry air in heated buildings, which can irritate the lungs, making them prone to infection. If you are constantly tired, catch colds easily, or are plagued with minor infections, try to identify your allergies.

Eat yogurt—People who regularly eat live-active culture yogurt appear to have stronger immune systems. Researchers from the University of California at Davis assigned three groups of volunteers either to consume a daily 450 gram (about 2 cups) serving of low-fat, live-active yogurt; yogurt without any active cultures; or no yogurt at all for four months. The results? Blood tests that analyzed white blood cells from the participants found that the people in the live-active yogurt group produced far more *gamma interferon,* a protein that boosts the immune response, than those who consumed the yogurt with no active cultures, or none at all.

Reduce stress—Stress is one of the greatest threats to the immune system. Exercise, especially outdoors, is a good stress reliever. Learn ways to monitor and control stressful situations; consider biofeedback, meditation, and yoga.

The body is self-healing and, very often, within a few days it will cure whatever is ailing us. If symptoms do not begin to disappear within a few days, see a physician; sometimes the cause of a weakened immune system is the result of an undiagnosed asymptomatic infection that a doctor can help you identify and treat.

Earl's Rx

This is my personal immune enhancing regimen.

Zinc: One 15–50 mg. capsule or tablet daily.

Betacarotene: One 25,000 IU capsule daily.

Vitamin E: One 400 IU capsule daily, dry form preferred.

Vitamin C: Two (500 mg.) calcium ascorbate tablets daily. (Calcium ascorbate is the form of vitamin C best tolerated by the stomach.)

Astralagus: One to three 400 mg. capsules daily.

Echinacea: One 500 mg. capsule one to three times daily for two weeks. Discontinue for two weeks, then resume. (If echinacea is overused, the beneficial effects will wear off.)

Gluthathione: One 500–1000 mg. capsule daily on an empty stomach.

Melatonin: One 1 mg. capsule or tablet daily, at bedtime. A sublingual form is available.

DHEA: One 25 mg. tablet or capsule daily.

Impotence

Some 25 million American men suffer from some form of impotence.

I mpotence is defined as the inability to maintain an erection adequate for satisfactory sexual performance. Although men don't necessarily like to talk about it, impotence is a very common problem, starting at around middle age. According to the Massachusetts Male Aging Study, a study of 1290 men between the ages of forty and seventy, about half of all men at one time or another experience a bout of impotence. The likelihood of suffering from impotence dramatically increases with age: At age forty, about 5 percent of all men are completely impotent, but that number reaches 15 percent by age seventy.

The good news is that most cases of impotence are completely preventable simply by maintaining a healthy lifestyle. For example, we know from the Massachusetts Aging Study that men who smoke are much more likely to become impotent than non smokers. We also know that coronary heart disease (atherosclerosis) and diabetes (which can lead to circulatory disorders) greatly increase the odds of becoming impotent. The reason is simple: In order to maintain an erection, the blood must flow freely to the penis. If the arteries delivering blood to the penis become clogged due to atherosclerosis, it can become impossible to maintain an erection. High blood pressure also dramatically increases the likelihood of impotence, for two reasons. First, high blood pressure can have a detrimental effect on circulation. Second, many of the medications used to lower blood pressure can interfere with either sexual desire or the ability to maintain an erection. In sum, by practicing a heart-healthy lifestyle it may be possible to avoid becoming impotent. (Heart disease, diabetes, and high blood pressure are covered in greater detail in separate chapters.)

Here are some supplements that can help men to maintain a vigorous, healthy sex life.

Natural Hormones

DHEA—In an attempt to find the cause of impotence among the men in their study, the researchers of the Massachusetts Male Aging Study checked the levels of various hormones in all men to see if there was any difference in impotent men. You might expect that impotent men would have lower levels of the primary male sex hormone, *testosterone*, but that was not the case. In fact, of the seventeen hormones measured, only one was noticeably lower in impotent men, and that hormone was DHEA. In fact, as levels of DHEA declined, the rate of impotency increased.

DHEA (short for *dehyroepiandrosterone*) is a hormone produced by the adrenal glands in both men and women that declines as we age. By age forty, we have half the amount of DHEA that we did at age twenty. In some people, the levels of DHEA drop even more precipitously. Why would low levels of DHEA contribute to impotence? There are several possible answers. DHEA is converted into testosterone in the body, and testosterone controls libido in both men and women. Therefore, it is possible that DHEA may have a sex-enhancing effect that helps men to maintain an erection. In addition, earlier studies have linked low levels of DHEA in men to an increased risk of heart disease. As I mentioned earlier, having heart disease greatly increases the likelihood that a man may develop impotence.

Since there have not been any clinical studies on DHEA and impotency, I must rely on anecdotal reports of men who take DHEA that it does improve libido and sexual performance. Until recently, DHEA was only available by prescription. It is now available over the counter at natural food stores.

Vitamins

Vitamin E—This vitamin not only improves circulation throughout the body, but it is a powerful antioxidant that can lower blood cholesterol and prevent atherosclerosis. Every man should take vitamin E either by itself or as part of an antioxidant complex. (If you are taking a blood thinner, check with your doctor before taking vitamin E.)

Betacarotene—Betacarotene (also called *provitamin A*) is converted into vitamin A as the body needs it. Vitamin A provides the raw material from which sex hormones are produced, and it is essential that we maintain high levels of vitamin A in our body. Vitamin A supplements can be toxic at very high doses; I recommend taking betacarotene, since the body will not produce more vitamin A than it needs.

Minerals

Zinc—This mineral is essential for the production of testosterone; low levels in men have been associated with infertility. (Zinc also helps to keep the prostate healthy. An enlarged prostate is a very common problem among middle-aged men, and can have a damping effect on a man's sex life. (See "Prostate Gland Enlargement," p. 234.)

Manganese—This mineral helps to produce two chemicals in the brain critical for sexual arousal: dopamine and acetylcholine.

Herbs

Ginkgo biloba—Ginkgo is *the* herb for good circulation; I believe that a ginkgo supplement is a must for every man. At least one study has shown that men who suffered from impotency due to circulatory problems were greatly helped by taking ginkgo supplements.

Yohimbe—The herb yohimbe is a much weaker version of the prescription drug yohimbine, which is often prescribed for impotence. The stronger yohimbine has been proven to be effective in many men, but it can have some serious side effects. The over-the-counter herb is safe, and many men find it to be helpful.

Personal Advice

Avoid alcohol—When it comes to sex, alcohol is a double-edged sword. Although alcohol can relax you, it can also inhibit erection and ejaculation in men. Chronic alcohol abuse can damage the nerves in the penis, rendering a man impotent.

Diabetics beware—If you are diabetic, be careful to maintain normal blood-sugar levels. There is evidence that elevated blood-sugar levels can cause nerve damage that can interfere with erection.

Earl's Rx

DHEA: One 25–50 mg. capsule daily. (DHEA should not be taken by anyone under forty. Men over fifty can take 50 mg. daily.)

Vitamin E: One 400 IU capsule daily; dry form is preferred because it is better absorbed by the body.

Betacarotene: One 6 mg. or 10,000 IU capsule daily.

Zinc: One 15–60 mg. capsule or tablet daily.

Manganese: Up to 9 mg. daily. (Manganese is often included in a multivitamin supplement, so if you are taking one, read the label. You may be getting enough of this mineral.)

Ginkgo biloba: One 60 mg. capsule or tablet daily.

Yohimbe: One to three 500 mg. capsules daily.

Indigestion

Over-the-counter drugs designed to relieve indigestion are a multibillion-dollar industry.

You can't turn on the television or radio without seeing a commercial for yet another new over-the-counter drug that is designed to "cure" indigestion. If you were to believe these commercials, it would appear as though everyone suffers from indigestion, and that the only way to treat this problem was with a battery of drugs. Nothing could be further from the truth! When it comes to indigestion, I believe that natural remedies are better, gentler, and every bit as effective as the arsenal of heavily advertised drugs.

Digestion is the process by which food is broken down to a form that may be readily absorbed from the stomach by the cells of the body. Digestion actually begins in the mouth when food is chewed, and when enzymes in saliva begin to break down food into smaller components. The masticated food passes through the esophagus to the stomach, where it is liquefied by a mixture of hydrochloric acid and pepsin, which is secreted by the stomach wall.

Gastric-acid secretion is a vital step in digestion and assimilation, particularly of proteins and minerals. Too much or too little can have negative effects on the digestion of food and consequently on your health.

As we age, our bodies produce less hydrochloric acid, which is essential for the digestion of food. As a result, people over fifty often develop chronic indigestion, which is characterized by gas and bloating after eating. To make matters worse, people with this problem often turn to over-the-counter antacids which, of course, will not help and can even hurt because reduction in the amount of acid is what is causing the problem in the first place!

In some cases, of course, indigestion may be caused by too much acid, but that does not give you carte blanche to take antacids indiscriminately. A better approach would be to avoid eating foods that stimulate acid production (such as coffee, chocolate, and cola drinks) and to eat small, frequent meals as opposed to one large meal.

If you have chronic indigestion, see your doctor to determine the cause. Symptoms of indigestion, including gas and bloating, could be a sign of another problem, such as gall-bladder disease or even a ulcer. If you and your physician have determined that your digestive discomfort is not due to other medical problems, you may want to try some natural remedies. I guarantee that they will make you feel better!

Herbs

Bromelain—Have a piece of fresh pineapple for dessert! Pineapple contains bromelain, which is a protein-digesting enzyme group that promotes good digestion and assists the absorption of nutrients from foods and supplements. Some people with too much stomach acid may find fresh pineapple to be irritating. For these people, I recommend bromelain in chewable tablets.

Betaine hydrochloric acid—This is a supplement made from beets. For people who produce too little HCL, it can help to get the digestive juices flowing.

Herbals teas—These infusions are excellent for digestion problems. Anise, fennel, catnip, chamomile, and peppermint teas are particularly soothing for an agitated stomach. One study shows that chamomile relaxes the digestive tract as well as the opium based drug papaverine. Anise has been used for more than 2,000 years for many ailments, including upset stomach and flatulence.

Cinnamon, ginger, and clove—These spices are not only delicious additions to cookies and pudding, they also help break down fats in your digestive system, probably by boosting digestive enzyme activity.

Add some herbs to your salad!—Dill, oregano, and fennel not only help relax digestive-tract muscles, they are also antifoaming agents that help prevent the formation of intestinal gas and inhibit the growth of several bacteria that attack the intestinal tract.

Papaya—This fruit has been used by Caribbean Indians for centuries for many medicinal remedies and as a digestive aid. They were onto something! The most important digestive enzyme in papaya is *papain*, which is similar to the human digestive enzyme *pepsin*. It also contains other enzymes which break down milk proteins and help digest starches. Today papaya extract is the active ingredient in most commercial meat tenderizers.

Personal Advice

Fresh fruits and vegetables and grains and cereal contain fiber which is essential for healthy colon and bowel function. Eat a diet that is high in those foods and relatively low in the more difficult to digest meat and fatty products.

Eating several small meals throughout the day instead of a large meal at night will help allow the body to properly digest food. Pay attention to the foods that cause gastrointestinal distress, and try eliminating those foods from your diet to see if your condition improves. Include some form of physical exercise in your daily regimen.

Before automatically reaching for the bottle of antacid, remember the cause of your distress may not necessarily be *too much* acid, but can also be caused by *too little*. Before self-diagnosing, check with your doctor or natural healer.

Earl's Rx

For digestive woes, try the following.

For too little HCL:

Betaine HCL: One 500 mg. tablet of betaine HCL with food, along with a complete multiple-digestive-enzyme formula (in capsule and tablet form) one half hour after eating a large meal. Take with a full glass of filtered water.

Bromelain: Chew one to two tablets after meals.

For too much HCL:

Papaya Tablets: Chewable papaya tablets can be taken after meals. I prefer them to antacids.

Kidney Stones

Kidney stones are a very common malady, affecting 10 percent of all men and 3 percent of all women.

The kidneys are incredibly hard-working organs that remove excess waste and fluid from the blood. Kidney stones are obstructions that can cause inflammation and damage by interfering with urination. Kidney stones can be extremely painful and there are few successful medical treatments. When it comes to kidney stones, prevention can go a long way.

Minerals

Calcium—Kidney stones are composed of two primary substances, calcium and *oxalate,* a chemical found in plants that binds with minerals such as calcium. Foods that are high in oxalates include beets, strawberries, chocolate, nuts, and tea. For years, doctors have been advising patients who suffer from kidney stones to severely curb their intake of calcium and to limit their intake of foods high in oxalates. On the surface, this makes sense, since both of these substances are the primary ingredients in kidney stones. However, a recent study performed at the Harvard School of Public Health found that at least half of this advice was wrong. Researchers studied the diets of more than fifty thousand middle-aged men. Much to the researchers' surprise, those who ate a diet rich in calcium were 34 percent *less likely* to develop calcium containing kidney stones those men on low-calcium diets. In other words, contrary to popular belief, a high-calcium diet appeared to protect against stones!

How could such a long-held theory be so off mark? Here's the likely explanation. In reality, it appears as if the extra oxalate—not extra calcium—may be the culprit. As I mentioned earlier, oxalate binds with calcium, but what happens if there is not enough calcium to which it can bind? Under normal circumstances, oxalate should bind with calcium and be absorbed in the intestinal tract. When there is not enough calcium, however, the oxalate is excreted through the urinary tract, which means that it must pass through the kidneys, where it can form those troublesome stones.

This leads to the next question: Is there any value to restricting the amount of oxalate in your diet? The experts say that if you are prone to kidney stones, it makes sense not to gorge on foods that are high in oxalates, but that eating them in moderation should do no harm.

Potassium—The same study that discovered that calcium actually prevents kidney stones also revealed another important new fact: Men with the highest intake of fruits and vegetables had half the risk of developing kidney stones as men who did not eat as much of these foods. The reason? Researchers speculate that another important mineral, potassium, which is abundant in fruits and vegetables, may also help to prevent the formation of kidney stones.

Magnesium—This mineral can help to dissolve small kidney stones before they become major problems.

Vitamins

B6—For years, I have been recommending that people with a tendency to form kidney stones take extra vitamin B6, which is not only a natural diuretic (it promotes urination, thus flushing out the kidneys), but seems to actually help to dissolve stones.

Herbs

Uva ursi—This herb, which is often used for urinary tract infections, is also a mild diuretic and is excellent for maintaining the health of the urinary-tract system.

Personal Advice

Water! Water! Water!—It is essential to drink eight to ten glasses of water daily to flush out the kidneys.

Diet tips—Eat five servings a day of fruits and vegetables to make sure that you are getting enough potassium. Foods rich in potassium include dried apricots, yogurt (also an excellent source of calcium), orange juice, potatoes, lima beans, and, of course, bananas.

Earl's Rx

Calcium and magnesium: Take 1000 mg. of calcium and 500 mg. of magnesium daily.

Potassium: One 99 mg. tablet up to three times daily.

Vitamin B6: Take 50 mg. of vitamin B6 up to three times daily.

Macular Degeneration

7.5 million American adults will suffer loss of vision due to macular degeneration by the year 2020.

M acular degeneration is the leading cause of irreversible blindness for people over the age of sixty. What is particularly frightening about this disease is the fact that there is no known treatment. There is a ray of hope, however, that antioxidants may help to prevent or lessen the severity of vision loss.

Macular degeneration is due to the destruction of a particular part of the eye that is critical for normal vision. The eye is an exquisitely designed machine that controls one of the most complicated processes in the body—the ability to see. When we look at something, the image is focused on the retina, the innermost layer of cells at the rear of the eyeball. Special cells in the retina translate light energy into nerve impulses that send images to the brain every time they are stimulated by light. The brain perceives these images as sight. The *macula* is a small dimple on the retina that is responsible for fine vision, the kind that is used for tasks such as writing, sewing, and distinguishing color. Damage to the macula can severely impair the ability to see; vision may get blurry, straight objects may appear bent, or a dark spot may appear in the field of vision. Eventually, victims of macular degeneration may lose all central vision.

The precise cause of macular degeneration is unknown, but many researchers suspect that it may be due to damage by free radicals, those unstable oxygen molecules that can wreak havoc on so many other parts of the body. Although still unproven, this theory makes sense. The eye is constantly exposed to ultraviolet light, which we know triggers the formation of free radicals on the skin and is the leading cause of skin cancer. In fact, the outer retina is rich in polyunsaturated fatty acids, which are especially prone to oxidative damage. The eye has its own defense system against free radicals—an arsenal of antioxidants including enzymes such as superoxide dismustase (SOD), glutathione peroxidase, and catalase (which work with zinc and copper), and vitamins such as C, E, and betacarotene. As we age, however, our body's natural defense system against free radicals weakens, and blood levels of important antioxidants drop. In fact, in a study published in the *Journal of the American Opto-*

metric Association (December 1993), researchers found that twenty-six out of twenty-eight patients with macular degeneration were deficient in at least one important antioxidant, and that twenty-one had deficiencies in at least two antioxidants. Researchers asked: Could replacing these antioxidants with supplements help strengthen our eyes' ability to ward off the destructive effects of free radicals? Here is what they discovered.

Vitamins

Carotenoids—A nationwide study of more than 850 people conducted by the Massachusetts Eye and Ear Infirmary in Boston and published in the *Journal of the American Medical Association* found that those who ate foods rich in carotenoids had half the estimated risk of developing age-related macular degeneration than those whose diets fell short. Interestingly, betacarotene, the best-known of the carotenoids, did not appear to be a major player in the macular degeneration story. Two other carotenoids (lutein and zeaxanthin) appeared to offer the most protection against macular degeneration; they are found primarily in dark leafy vegetables such as spinach and collard greens. High concentrations of lutein and zeaxanthin are also found in the yellow pigment in the macula of the eye, and researchers believe that these nutrients may screen out particular light rays that promote oxidative damage. (Both carotenoids are available in supplement form.)

Vitamin C—In a study of more than 2,100 people between the ages of forty-three and eighty-six, researchers found that those who took vitamin supplements were much less likely to develop macular degeneration than those who did not. In particular, those who took vitamin C showed a decrease in early macular degeneration. This is not surprising. In addition to being an important antioxidant in its own right, vitamin C raises the blood levels of an important antioxidant, glutathione, which is found in many cells, including those of the eye.

Minerals

Zinc—Researchers put two facts together and came up with zinc. Here's how. Zinc deficiency is common in older adults, and zinc is essential for the metabolic function of some cell layers in the retina. Could zinc somehow play a role in macular degeneration? Yes, according to researchers at Louisiana State University. In their ground-breaking study headed by David A. Newsome, M.D., some 151 patients with macular degeneration were given either a placebo or 100 mg. of oral zinc twice daily, considerably more than the RDA of 15 mg. The results: after a follow-up period of one to two years, those taking zinc had significantly less loss of vision than the placebo group. Another year-long study involving pigs showed that those receiving a low-zinc diet were found to have degenerative changes in the eye similar to those found in the early stages of macular degeneration.

Herbs

Ginkgo biloba—In Europe, extract of ginkgo biloba has been used in the treatment of macular degeneration. Ginkgo is a potent antioxidant.

Personal Advice

Quit smoking—Smokers are at a greater risk of developing macular degeneration than nonsmokers. Why? Probably because each puff of smoke promotes the formation of free radicals that can destroy the delicate eye tissue.

Watch your diet—People with high cholesterol are at a greater risk of developing macular degeneration than people with normal levels of cholesterol. Why? Probably because high cholesterol causes clogged arteries, which can impair the flow of blood to the eyes.

Earl's Rx

These potent antioxidants should help to keep you seeing clearly!

Antioxidant multivitamin with minerals and B-complex: Two tablets daily (one in the morning, one at night) with food.

Gingko biloba: Three 60 mg. capsules or tablets daily.

Grapeseed and green-tea extract combination: Two to three tablets daily.

Memory Loss

Loss of short-term memory is a common occurrence past age fifty.

Hot, new, over-the-counter supplements can help you stay smart and sharp!

Does this sound familiar? You're introduced to someone at a party and, within a few seconds, you're embarrassed to admit that you've already forgotten his name! Although this can happen to anyone at any time, it is much more likely to happen at around age fifty, when nearly everyone begins to show signs of short-term memory loss.

Short-term memory involves the part of the brain used to recall recently acquired facts, like a new phone number or a new address. By their sixth decade, most people will experience a more noticeable decline in short-term memory and alertness. This doesn't mean that we are all destined to suffer from severe memory-loss disorders such as Alzheimer's or senility—not at all. It does mean, however, that about 75 percent of all older people will have some difficulty in remembering.

Memory is the process of both storing and retrieving information. There are different types of memory; some forms of memory involve retaining great amounts of knowledge, such as a new language, or concepts like mathematical theorems. Other types of memory may involve the recollection of a single experience or bit of information. Any kind of memory loss, however, can be very annoying, and can make you feel older than your years.

The loss of memory in some people may be due to the fact that an older brain may not produce the same quantity and quality of chemicals—neurotransmitters—involved in memory function. There are several reasons this happens:

- The blood supply to the brain could be impeded by atherosclerosis or other circulatory problems.

- Medication could be interfering with brain function.

- Poor diet could be causing nutritional deficiencies, starving the brain of important nutrients.

* Emotional problems such as the loss of a spouse, stress, and even boredom may also interfere with brain function.

An improved diet, supplements, and some changes in lifestyle may help keep your memory sharp.

Vitamins

Vitamin B1 (Thiamine)—Studies have shown that low levels of B1 can cause subtle changes in brain function among older people that could contribute to memory loss. Good food sources of B1 include brewer's yeast, unrefined cereal grains, pompano fish, sunflower seeds, ham, and peanuts.

Folic acid—Folic acid may prevent memory loss by helping to maintain normal levels of *homocysteine,* an amino acid found in the body. According to a recent study performed by the Agriculture Research Service of the U.S. Department of Agriculture, researchers found a strong correlation between high blood levels of homocysteine and the loss of memory and the ability to learn that often accompanies depression in the elderly.

A preliminary study of depressed patients by researchers at Human Nutrition Research Center on Aging at Tufts University, Boston, found that high levels of homocysteine have the potential to damage the brain by two routes. First, by increasing the risk for cardiovascular disease, which can impair blood function to the brain. Second, homocysteine is converted to an amino acid that stimulates brain cell receptors at normal levels, but can cause the cells to self-destruct at excess levels. Blood analyses of twenty-seven elderly patients showed that homocysteine levels were highest in the patients with vascular disease and, in those free of vascular disease, homocysteine levels were highest in the patients who scored lowest on cognitive tests.

Good food sources of folic acid include dark-green leafy vegetables, sunflower seeds, wheat germ, liver, and peanuts. Folic acid is now being added to packaged dry cereals, and is also available in supplement form.

Vitamin B12—Folic acid is interdependent with vitamin B12; both are required by rapidly dividing cells, and a deficiency of one will lead to a deficiency of the other. For many people over age sixty, a lack of vitamin B12 may be responsible for certain neurologic symptoms ranging from weakness, lack of balance, mood changes, disorientation, and memory loss. Doctors at the University Hospital of Maastricht in the Netherlands have found that otherwise healthy people with lower blood levels of B12 don't perform as well on mental tests as people with higher levels.

This deficiency may not necessarily be due to the fact that people are not eating enough foods rich in this vitamin, but because up to 40 percent of people over age sixty have atrophic gastritis, which means that their stomachs no longer produce enough hydrochloric acid for the body to effectively use the B12 they are getting from food. This condition is easy enough to treat with supplements of hydrochloric acid but, unfortunately, since there are no apparent symptoms, the deficiency is not usually picked up in a routine exam. Acid levels can be determined by certain tests; check with your physician.

Choline—Choline has been identified as being a key to memory function. Researchers suspect that choline can help to retard the effects of normal aging on the brain from midlife on. Choline's benefits are twofold: First, it is utilized by the brain to make *acetylcholine*, a neurotransmitter involved in memory function, second, it may keep nerve-cell membranes, including the *synapses* (the communication points between brain cells) intact, which enables brain cells to "talk" to each other and share information.

As we age, we begin to produce less acetylcholine, or the acetylcholine that is produced is less efficient, which may be why many older people become forgetful. The utilization of choline in the body depends on several other nutrients, principally vitamin B12, folic acid, and the amino acid L-carnitine.

The body uses L-carnitine to produce the enzyme *acetyl-L-carnitine transferase*, which boosts choline metabolism and releases acetylcholine in the brain. According to the results of an Italian study published in November 1991 *Neurology* (November 1991), 2 grams of carnitine taken daily for a year improved the attention span, long-term memory, and verbal ability of Alzheimer's patients. It is believed that L-carnitine can also help less serious forms of memory loss.

Good food sources of choline include eggs, soybeans, cabbage, peanuts, and cauliflower. Choline is also available in supplements.

Mighty Minerals

Zinc and iron—Taken separately, these minerals appear to boost memory. Researchers at the University of Texas gave 30 mg. supplements of either iron or zinc to twenty-six women who were deficient in those minerals. After replenishing their zinc and iron, the researchers found that the women's standard memory scores increased by 10 to 20 percent.

Iron—Iron deficiency has been shown to lower test scores by college students. Students at Penn State who were found to be deficient in iron significantly increased their test scores after three months of taking iron supplements. Now that people are cutting back on iron-rich red meat, they need to be especially careful about getting iron in other forms. Good food sources of iron are pork, oysters, clams, chicken, and turkey. Iron supplements should only be taken in cases of iron-deficient anemia.

Antioxidants

Free radicals are unstable oxygen molecules that are normal byproducts of the cells use of oxygen. Free radicals bind readily with other molecules and, when they do, they give off energy that can damage cells within the body. Brain tissue is particularly vulnerable to oxidative damage, and many researchers believe that over time, free radicals can effect brain function.

The body uses antioxidants to defend itself against these potentially harmful unstable molecules. While some antioxidants are enzymes produced by the body, we get others from the foods we eat, and through supplements such as vitamins C and E.

Researchers studying the protective effects of antioxidants on the brain at the University of California in San Francisco found some antioxidant enzymes such as super oxide disutase (SOD) effectively reduced free-radical damage caused by inadequate blood flow to the brain due to stroke or arteriosclerosis.

New and Over-the-Counter

A new hormone, *pregnenolone,* is now being sold over-the-counter and is reputed to be the most potent memory-enhancing agent to date. In animal studies, only a few molecules of this hormone vastly improved the memory of mice. But it's not just mice who have shown improvement on this remarkable hormone. More than fifty years ago, pregnenolone was shown to enhance learning skills, elevate mood, and improve the job performance of factory workers and airline pilots. What's even more exciting is that researchers say that this hormone is safe, and has no known side effects!

Herbs

Club moss tea—This tea has been found to contain natural memory-enhancing compounds. Researchers at the Shanghai Institute of Materia Medica reported they had isolated two compounds from club moss tea, huperzine A and huperzine B which, according to laboratory tests, helped to improve learning, memory retrieval, and memory retention.

Gingko biloba—The leaves of the ginkgo tree are a rich source of bioflavonoids and other components which have many medicinal properties.

Ginkgo has been shown in animal studies to increase the levels of *dopamine*, a chemical found in the brain that improves the body's ability to transmit information.

A study reported in the *British Journal of Clinical Pharmacology* (1992) found that 120 to 160 mg. per day of ginkgo biloba extract given to volunteers for at least four to six weeks produced a positive effect on circulation to the brain. The volunteers experienced improved concentration, better memory, and less absentmindedness and confusion. Researchers believe that the herb may work by preventing damage from free radicals.

Gotu kola—This herb has been used in India and China for hundreds of years, where it is part of traditional herbal medicine. Recent studies show that gotu kola has a positive effect on the circulatory system by strengthening the veins and capillaries, thereby improving the flow of blood throughout the body, including to the brain.

Siberian ginseng—This form of ginseng has been known to ancient Chinese for more than three thousand years. There are many types of ginseng, but Siberian ginseng has long been valued by the Chinese for its value in increasing longevity, improving general health, and restoring memory.

Personal Advice

Watch your blood pressure—High blood pressure can cause memory loss. Once the blood pressure is normalized, however, the memory loss will stop. (See "High Blood Pressure," p. 156.)

Use It or Lose It—Some researchers believe that the memory centers of the brain can be tweaked much the way muscles can be pumped; that is, like a muscle, these memory centers will lose their efficiency if they are not used. One of the best mental exercises for maintaining an active mind is by flexing your creative muscles.

Often, as people age, they tend to depend more on stored knowledge than on new knowledge. But by expanding your creative interests into new areas, you will literally be flexing your mental muscles. Don't think retirement and old age is the end of creativity. It might be just the time to pursue a long-suppressed interest—writing, music lessons, volunteering, painting,—the list is endless. (You might ask your grandchildren to teach you how to play video games—there is evidence that involvement in a nonaerobic activity such as video games may also improve cognitive abilities of older people.)

Researchers at Mt. Sinai Medical School, N.Y., report that there is less mental decline in people who adapt easily to change, who like learning new things, and enjoy going to new places.

Move it or lose it!—Put down that remote control! There's a reason why getting up and out helps you to stay mentally alert. Researchers have found that physical inactivity is accompanied by electrical and chemical changes in the brain; there is a gradual winding down of brain-wave frequency and decreased levels of two neurotransmitters, dopamine and noradrenaline. Exercise reverses that decrease.

You don't have to become an Olympic athlete to take advantage of the benefits of exercise. Whatever activity you decide to do, whether it's walking, jogging, swimming, or golfing, the important thing is to do it regularly.

Watch the alcohol—It isn't difficult to understand that alcohol can impair mental function—try to remember your own telephone number after you've had one too many! But those who are habitual drinkers should be aware that alcohol ranks fourth as a cause of progressive dementia, with the heaviest drinkers most affected.

Control stress—Stress affects every part of the body, so it follows that stress can also affect the mind. In fact, some memory experts say that heavy stress is a big contributing factor to some forms of memory loss. Researchers at McGill University in Montreal checked the concentration of the stress hormone *cortisol* in the blood of 130 healthy volunteers age fifty-five to eighty-seven for five years. The results indicate that high amounts of cortisol correlate with subtle memory and attention problems.

Do anything you can to relieve stress, from facing what's causing the stress to meditation to exercise, especially yoga and biofeedback.

Be aware of the effects your medication has on your body. It's all too easy to prescribe drugs for the elderly in order to sedate, calm, or ease pain. The problem is that a mixture of sedatives, benzodiazepines, antidepressants, antihistamines, diuretics, heart medication, steroids, and tranquilizers, are among the most prescribed medications for the elderly.

Unfortunately, physicians don't always advise patients of the dangers of mixing drugs—and many times, several doctors are treating the same patient and may not even know what the others have prescribed. Take charge, ask questions, and always tell your physician what drugs you are taking.

There does not appear to be a direct relationship between memory loss and menopause. However, some of the problems associated with menopause are also associated with memory loss. These disturbances include insomnia, which is often a result of night sweats, fatigue, depression, and gastric distress.

Finally, get enough sleep. Numerous studies have documented that when you are sleep-deprived, you can't think or learn as well the next day.

Earl's Rx

Here is a good memory regimen.

Antioxidant-B-complex multivitamin: Special antioxidant formulas containing B-complex vitamins are now being sold in natural-food stores. This combination is essential for anyone with a flagging memory. Take one pill or capsule in the morning with food, and one in the evening with food.

Gingko biloba: Three 60 mg. pills or capsules daily.

Choline: There are three types of choline sold at natural food stores: phosphatidyl choline, phosphatidyl inositol, or phosphatidyl serine. As far as I'm concerned, they all do a good job and you should use whichever is easiest for you to find. Take one capsule two to three times daily.

Pregnenolone: One or two 50 mg. capsules daily.

Siberian ginseng: One capsule or tablet, twice daily.

Menopause

In the next 20 years, an estimated 40 million American women will reach the age of menopause.

Approximately 75 percent of women will experience hot flashes at some time during menopause.

Physical discomfort due to menopause can often be eased or eliminated with natural remedies.

M enopause, the end of menstruation, is caused by a decline in the production of two hormones, estrogen and progesterone, by the ovaries. In the United States, most women become menopausal, or experience their last menstrual cycle, at around age fifty-one.

Both estrogen and progsterone are known for their role in sexuality and reproduction, but both perform a wide range of other critical tasks in the body. For example, *estrogen* is involved in everything from maintaining normal cholesterol levels, building bone, and even in memory and learning. *Progesterone,* which is produced in both the ovaries and the adrenal glands, is also essential for bone formation, sex drive, and is a natural tranquilizer that helps women cope with stress.

At menopause the body's overall estrogen levels decline about 80 percent, and although the ovaries are no longer making estrogen, some estrogen is still being produced by the adrenal glands and fat tissue. Production of progesterone is virtually nil, and many women feel the loss of these hormones acutely.

The most apparent (and annoying) effects of reduced estrogen are hot flashes and insomnia. Ailments that some women develop as they age, and which most researchers attribute to the loss of these female hormones, include osteoporosis, tooth decay, cardiac disease, arthritis, increased cholesterol levels, and bone fractures.

Clearly, estrogen and progesterone play an important role in a woman's health and well-being. About 15 percent of all post-menopausal women take hormones (a combination of estrogen and progesterone) to replace the hormones they are no longer producing on their own. Hormone-replacement therapy has been shown to protect against heart disease and osteoporosis, two serious diseases, and can relieve the unpleasant symptoms of menopause. Many women who are on HRT say they feel better—*much* better—on hormones; and would not even consider stopping therapy.

But HRT is not for everyone. Although the benefits of hormone replacement are well-known, it has some drawbacks. These include possible increased risk of breast cancer, possible increase of the risk of gallbladder disease, weight gain, breast tenderness, uterine bleeding, and fluid retention.

Although researchers generally agree that hormone replacement therapy is safe when estrogen and progesterone are taken together, there are many women who may be good candidates for HRT but still prefer to use natural solutions to natural problems.

What to do? Look to natural sources of hormones, supplements, herbs, diet, and change in lifestyle.

Vitamins

Vitamin E—Vitamin E has been used for more than fifty years as a remedy for hot flashes. A potent antioxidant, vitamin E can also help to protect postmenopausal women against heart disease, the number-one killer of women. (See "Heart Disease," p. 142.)

Vitamin C—Vitamin C can help strengthen capillaries and lessen the effect of vasomotor disturbances that can cause those annoying hot flashes.

B complex—A multivitamin and mineral formula that contains all the major B vitamins is important to help control stress.

Calcium and vitamin D—Calcium is the most abundant mineral in the human body. Roughly 99 percent of the body's calcium is found in the teeth and bones. Calcium is instrumental in muscle contraction, blood clotting, and maintenance of cell membranes, and plays a critical role in the normal functioning of the heart. This is important because heart disease in women increases after menopause.

One of the most devastating effects of menopause is bone loss, which leads to fractures, spine curvature, and tooth loss. (See "Osteoporosis," p. 212.) Calcium supplements are advised for menopausal women, although it is beneficial to begin sufficient calcium intake at an early age.

Good food sources of calcium include low-fat milk and yogurt, fortified juice and cereals, salmon and sardines with bones, and molasses. Vitamin D increases calcium absorption in the body, and magnesium appears to regulate the flow of calcium between cells.

Avoid cola drinks that contain phosphate: This mineral saps calcium from the body. Caffeine and alcohol can also decrease calcium absorption.

Magnesium—This mineral is essential for strong bones and is also heart-healthy. In one important study of women with mild high blood pressure sponsored by the Netherlands Heart Foundation, magnesium supplements reduced blood pressure in women not taking other medication.

In addition, magnesium can help to prevent insulin resistance, that is, the inability to use insulin efficiently to turn glucose into energy. As a result of insulin resistance, glucose levels rise, which can lead to diabetes and heart disease.

Phytoestrogens

Soy—*Phytoestrogens* are plant compounds that are converted during the normal digestive process into a form of very weak estrogen. Soybeans are rich in phytoestrogens, and although they may be thousands of times weaker than the body's steroidal hormones, they can still exert a powerful influence.

Many researchers believe that phytoestrogens may help manipulate the hormonal environment in a favorable way. They are structurally similar to the estrogen that is produced by the body—so similar, in fact, that they can literally fool cells into thinking they are the real thing. Although phytoestrogens are far weaker than natural estrogen, if they occur in high enough concentrations, they can out-compete the natural estrogens for binding spots on estrogen-sensitive cells.

Soy products such as soy milk, tofu, and soy flour might also improve the blood-cholesterol balance which sometimes increases in post-menopausal women, and offset some of the more distressing affects of a drop in estrogen such as vaginal dryness, night sweats, insomnia, and fatigue.

Herbs

Siberian ginseng—Fatigue is one of the most common complaints of menopause. Siberian ginseng, which is similar to Asian ginseng, is an excellent tonic that helps improve energy levels. All forms of ginseng are rich in phytoestrogens, which can help to relieve menopausal symptoms. (In rare cases, ginseng can stimulate the uterine lining causing menstrual-type bleeding, in a manner similar to real estrogen. If you experience any irregular bleeding during menopause, be sure to contact your physician or natural healer and let her know that you are using ginseng.)

Dong quai—For centuries, Chinese women have used dong quai for a wide range of female gynecological complaints. Modern researchers confirm its usefulness against acute symptoms of menopause caused by hormonal changes. Rich in minerals and vitamins including A, B12, and E, dong quai has also been used to treat insomnia, one of the more debilitating effects of menopause.

Vitex—Also known as *chaste tree berries*, this plant is reputed to stabilize hormone levels. Vitex is found in many herbal formulas designed to treat menopausal symptoms.

Anise, fennel, licorice root, and red clover—These herbs contain phytoestrogens, which may account for their traditional use as a milk promoter in nursing mothers. Although each has only mild estrogenic activity, they may help ease some of the discomforts of menopause, especially when added to other phytoestrogenic herbs and foods.

Foods rich in phytoestrogens include alfalfa, apples, barley, carrots, cherries, chick peas, garlic, green beans, oats, peas, potatoes, rice, rye, wheat, and, especially, yams.

Natural progesterone—Body creams containing Mexican yam root are a nonprescription source for a natural, nontoxic, progesterone. These over-the-counter progesterone creams can relieve mild menopausal symptoms for many women. In addition, progesterone creams may, like estrogen, protect against osteoporosis. In fact, recent studies demonstrate that progesterone can halt the loss of bone at least as well as estrogen. We know that estrogen can slow the loss of bone after menopause, reducing the risk of fracture by 50 percent, but estrogen is unable to stimulate the formation of new bone. According to researcher Dr. Jerilynn C. Prior, of the University of British Columbia in Vancouver, who has performed some ground-breaking studies on the role of progesterone in the maintenance of bone, progesterone may be able to do what estrogen cannot, that is, it can actually help to grow *new bone*.

For example, in animal studies, progesterone administered with or without estrogen has been shown not only to stop bone loss, but to enhance new bone formation. In fact, some of Dr. Prior's animal studies have shown that there are progesterone receptors or binding sites on *osteoblasts*, the cells that build bone. The assumption is, if progesterone goes to these bone-building sites, it must do so for a purpose.

Dr. John R. Lee is a California physician who is a well-known proponent of natural progesterone. For three years, Dr. Lee followed the progress of one hundred postmenopausal women, aged thirty-eight to eighty-three, who were at risk of developing osteoporosis. In addition to putting the women on a healthy diet, which included supplemental calcium and vitamin D, Dr. Lee prescribed estrogen to women who could take it, along with a natural progesterone cream that was applied daily during the last two weeks of estrogen use each month. To women who could not take estrogen, he prescribed a natural progesterone cream applied twelve days a month. (This is in keeping with the natural ebb and flow of estrogen and progesterone during the menstrual cycle.) The women were instructed to get regular exercise, forbidden to smoke, and told to limit their alcohol intake. At the end of three years, bone-density studies of sixty-three of the patients revealed that the regimen had not only slowed down the osteoporosis, but that it had reversed it. These women had an increase in bone density, which indicated that the patients had not only stopped losing bone, but were actually gaining new bone. Dr. Lee notes that although some patients improved more than others, all the patients improved. Surprisingly, according to Dr. Lee, the patients taking the estrogen/progesterone combination did not fare any better than the patients taking progesterone alone. Dr. Lee, who has written several excellent books on natural progesterone, has come to the conclusion that osteoporosis is actually a disease of progesterone deficiency and that estrogen plays a minor role in osteoporosis, if any.

Personal Advice

Don't wait until you reach menopause to start taking care of yourself. Start early on a lifelong course of good health habits. Eat a balanced diet, rich in calcium and low in fat. Whole natural foods, which include greens like watercress, dandelion greens, chickweed, and various types of seaweed, are all rich in calcium. Get sufficient vitamin D from low-fat dairy products, vitamin supplements and outdoor activities to help your body absorb the calcium.

Don't smoke, and limit alcohol and caffeine. Most important, include physical activity or exercise in your daily routine. Drink plenty of water to counteract the drying effect of loss of estrogen. Get enough restful sleep and try to reduce stress. Meditation, yoga, and deep breathing are good stress relievers.

Earl's Rx

These supplements work well for menopausal symptoms.

Vitamin E: One or two capsules daily (400 IU) of the dry form.

Vitamin C: Take 1000 mg. daily of calcium ascorbate.

B-complex (with B6): One 50 mg. tablet or capsule daily.

Calcium and vitamin D: Take 1200 mg. calcium with 400 IU vitamin D.

Magnesium: Take 500 mg. chelated magnesium.

Dong quai: Two tablets or capsules daily. Dong quai is included in many menopause herbal formulas.

Siberian ginseng: One to three capsules daily.

Natural progesterone cream: Typically, women use natural progesterone cream for twelve days out of every month. The amount of cream that is normally used is ¼ to ½ teaspoon applied twice daily (morning and night) to the abdomen, back, shoulders, neck, arms, and face.

Muscle Strain

More Americans of all ages are participating in fitness programs than at any other time in history.

The most common form of injury associated with exercise and sports activities is muscle strain.

The human body has about seven-hundred different muscles and sometimes, after a tough workout, it may feel as if all seven hundred of them are screaming out in pain!

Muscle consists of threads, or *muscle fibers*, supported by connective tissue, which act by contraction. Muscles that are overworked or weak to begin with can tire, which produces the aches and pains that we associate with muscle strain. When a muscle is strained or injured, it is usually a result of inflammation.

Weekend athletes and those who exercise sporadically—especially those who fail to warm up and stretch their muscles before taking that long hike or bike ride—are most prone to suffer from muscle strain.

There are several simple things you can do to help reduce the swelling. Applying ice to the area, resting the muscle, and elevating the injured limb, will all help.

But the actual repair of the injured muscle is done by the cells of the body, and they need extra fuel to meet the challenge. The following supplements can be helpful in promoting healing and relieving some of the discomfort.

Vitamins

Bioflavonoids (flavonoids)—These chemicals are found in grapes, onions, red peppers, and citrus fruits, which work together with vitamin C and other enzymes and nutrients to help strengthen capillary walls.They have been successfully used to treat bruises and sprains.

In a study conducted at San Jose College, the incidence of injuries from a variety of sports were reduced by 50 percent, and the rate of recovery from muscle injury was increased by 50 percent, in those athletes taking bioflavonoids and vitamin C.

Researchers at Louisiana State University recently showed that the number of muscle strains due to football injuries was reduced by 50 percent in those taking bioflavonoids and Vitamin C. Forty-eight football players took part in the study, and those using bioflavonoids and vitamin C had less bruising, and a faster recovery time for sprains.

Vitamin E— Although exercise is wonderful for your physical and mental wellbeing, there is one down side; all that huffing and puffing means that your body must consume more oxygen which, in turn, leads to the production of more free radicals. As I have mentioned before, free radicals can inflict significant damage to the cells of the body and, in fact, some of what we experience as muscle strain may be due to damage by free radicals. Vitamin E, one of nature's most potent antioxidants, appears to help to prevent at least some of the exercise-induced damage. In a double-blind study reported in *The American Journal of Physiology* (1993), researchers evaluated nine males age twenty-two to twenty-nine and twelve males fifty-five to seventy-four years of age, who consumed either 800 IU of vitamin E or a placebo daily.

All participants exercised at 75 percent of their maximum heart rate for 45 minutes. The men who received vitamin E showed reduced free-radical damage to the tissues, with the greatest protective effect seen in younger individuals.

Another study at the Human Nutrition Research Center on Aging at Tufts, showed that vitamin E may reduce some of the muscle damage that occurs during rigorous exercise by protecting cells from oxidation. Researchers studied 21 sedentary men: Half were given 800 IU of vitamin E for seven days prior to running downhill on a treadmill for 45 minutes, and half were given placebos. Those who received the vitamin E excreted significantly less of a byproduct of fat oxidation and had significantly lower blood levels of two substances that trigger inflammation.

Both these studies strongly suggest that taking vitamin E supplements before beginning exercise will produce less pain afterwards.

B-complex—Anytime your body is under stress—such as when you are undertaking vigorous exercise—you need to fortify yourself with additional B vitamins.

Herbs

Arnica ointment—Sold in natural-food stores, arnica ointment is excellent for overworked muscles but will irritate broken skin.

Eucalyptus ointment—An ointment made from the eucalyptus tree can help by promoting blood flow to the sore muscles, which produces a feeling of warmth.

White willow bark—I recommend this aspirinlike herbal compound for pain and inflammation.

Grapeseed extract—Rich in protective bioflavonoids, this supplement can help reduce inflammation.

Personal Advice

Easy does it!—The first consideration is so obvious that you probably already know what you need to do. It's just getting you to do what's good for you that's difficult. First, don't decide on the spur of the moment to engage in strenuous exercise without giving the endeavor some forethought. Stretching (but not overextending) muscles first is important. Begin an exercise or athletic program gradually, building to optimum capabilities over a period of time.

One of the most important things to do is to drink, even if you don't feel thirsty. Drink at least sixteen to twenty ounces of fluid two hours before exercising and another eight ounces 15 to 30 minutes afterwards. Sip four to six ounces every 15 to 20 minutes while exercising.

It is possible to lose two quarts of water during strenuous physical activity—unfortunately, you may not even feel thirsty, and the longer you go without replenishing fluids, the more difficult it is to reestablish your body's fluid balance.

If you plan to make regular physical activity part of your life (and everyone should partake in some kind of physical activity), increase the amount of raw foods you eat. This will help increase enzymatic action, which will help those overworked muscles to better repair themselves. Drink fresh juices and herbal teas. Avoid colas, white sugar, refined flour, and fried foods, which all increase body stress.

In addition to vitamin C and bioflavonoids, other anti-inflammatory agents include the B vitamins, especially B1, B2, B3, B5, B6, and B12.

Earl's Rx

If you suffer from muscle strain, try the following

Vitamin E: One 400 IU capsule, twice daily, dry form preferred.

B-complex: One 50 mg. capsule or tablet with each meal, up to three times daily.

White willow bark: One or two capsules, every three to four hours, as needed for pain.

Grapeseed extract: One 100 mg. capsule or tablet, two to three times daily.

Bioflavonoid complex: One 1000 mg. capsule, twice daily.

Nausea

Nausea can be due to a queasy stomach or a sign of a more serious problem.

In most cases, natural remedies are preferable to prescription medications.

Nearly everyone has experienced nausea at one time or another, but not everyone gets nauseated from the same things. Nausea is caused by a number of chemical changes in the body, and can be triggered by many different factors, ranging from motion to emotional upset to foul odors. It is still a mystery why some people seem to be born with sea legs and others can't ride the Staten Island Ferry without becoming seasick. Other people will become ill at the sight of blood or the smell of rotten food, while others are not at all affected. And one person's gourmet delight will turn someone else's stomach.

The way we experience nausea is also highly individual. For many people nausea is frequently accompanied by faintness, excess saliva, perspiration, and low blood pressure. Although in most cases nausea is not a sign of a serious problem, is can also be part of a group of symptoms that are warning signs for both heart attack and stroke. For women in particular, extreme nausea and flulike symptoms may be a sign of a heart attack, but this could also be true for men. Therefore, anyone who is at risk of heart disease or other serious ailments should check with their physician if they are experiencing any untoward symptoms.

Due to hormonal shifts in the body, about half of all women experience nausea during pregnancy and, for the same reason, many women are nauseated right before their periods.

Nausea is usually a passing symptom that will almost always go away by itself. In most cases, I recommend natural remedies for nausea because they are often as effective as some of the prescription antiemetic drugs, but they do not cause unnecessary side effects. The only exception to this rule, however, is in the case of cancer patients who are receiving chemotherapy; the kind of intense nausea they may experience can be so severe that stronger measures may be needed. Fortunately, there are some new antinausea drugs that have proven to be quite effective for these patients, and they are truly a godsend.

For most people, however, help with routine nausea may be as close as your pantry.

Herbs

Ginger—Ginger root has a long traditional history as an effective cure for nausea. Ancient Greek physicians knew about ginger's positive effects and, in more modern times, it was used by Queen Elizabeth I as a digestive aid. In one double-blind study reported in *The Lancet,* a British medical journal, ginger was more effective than the drug Dramamine in preventing nausea associated with motion sickness. Another study treated sixty women who had had major gynecological surgery with either ginger or a placebo. Those receiving ginger had fewer incidences of nausea, and those who received the placebo required larger doses of antinausea drugs to relieve their symptoms.

Chamomile tea—This tea has traditionally been used as a digestive aid. Chamomile oil appears to have a relaxing action on the smooth muscle lining of the digestive tract, making it an antispasmodic. Many people are allergic to chamomile, however, so if you have hayfever, I would recommend that you avoid it.

Basil—This green herb is more than a delicious addition to Italian food, it is an effective remedy for a variety of digestive disorders, including nausea, vomiting, and stomach cramps.

Caraway—These seeds are often used in baked goods, and are known for their mildly spicy, aromatic flavor. Brewed in a tea, caraway helps improve digestion, expel gas, and reduce nausea.

Other herbal remedies for upset stomach and nausea are ginger-root tea, peppermint tea, and cinnamon.

Vitamins

Vitamin B-complex with B6 can aid in digestion (B vitamins help to metabolize protein and fat) and there is anecdotal evidence that it can relieve chronic nausea.

Personal Advice

If you suffer from morning sickness during pregnancy, try starting your day with a strong cup of peppermint tea. If your symptoms are very severe, two ginger capsules may do the trick. (Check with your physician or natural healer before taking any medication during pregnancy.)

Earl's Rx

If you are suffering from nausea, try drinking a strong cup of peppermint tea, in addition to taking the following.

Ginger: One capsule three times daily. If you do not have ginger capsules, you can suck on a small piece of fresh ginger root.

B-complex: Three 50 mg. capsules with vitamin B6 daily with meals.

Obesity

Nearly one-third of all Americans are obese, that is, more than 20 percent above ideal body weight.

When it comes to weight loss, there is no "magic bullet," but the right nutrition, exercise, and supplements can help shed excess pounds, and more important, prevent them from coming back.

Obesity is a veritable epidemic in the western world; in the United States, more than 30 percent of all men and women are seriously overweight. What I find to be particularly alarming is the fact that nearly 25 percent of all teenagers are obese, which places them at very high risk of becoming obese adults.

Obesity is not merely a cosmetic problem; it is a serious health hazard. People who are obese are more prone to develop many diseases, including various forms of cancer, heart disease, diabetes, and arthritis, and are more likely to die at a younger age. Not only can obesity rob you of years of life, but it can have a profoundly negative impact on lifestyle. It is simply not possible to feel or act your best when you are carrying around all that excess baggage.

Weight creep—slow but steady weight gain through the years—is an even more common problem than obesity, and can also be detrimental to health. Even though they are not technically obese, millions of Americans weigh more than they should; in fact, a weight gain of a few pounds each year is fairly typical. Until recently, the standard weight guideline charts used by insurance companies actually allowed for a twenty-five pound weight gain during adulthood. Recent studies suggest, however, that this weight is not only not normal, but downright unhealthy. One ground-breaking study tracked the lifestyle and health of 115,000 registered nurses over a sixteen-year period. Based on this study, researchers concluded that even a moderate weight gain (defined as more than 22 pounds) after age eighteen greatly increased the risk of early death. Due to this study and others like it, insurance companies have revised their weight recommendations downward.

I am not suggesting, however, that everyone has to be stick thin or that we should emulate the unrealistic body types of high-fashion models, not at all. What I am saying is that it is critical for everyone to maintain a healthy, normal weight based on their body type and nutritional needs.

What is a healthy weight? There are many different formulas designed to determine the correct weight for each person, but I prefer to take a more individual approach. The new insurance company guidelines can help to give you a ballpark figure, and you can check how you rate vis-à-vis these charts when you have your annual physical. How you feel is of equal importance. If you are healthy and energetic and eat a sensible diet but are on the high end of the weight scale, you are probably at your correct weight and trying to cut back will be an exercise in frustration. If, however, you are on the high end of normal, or slightly above normal, but are sedentary, eat a poor diet and look and feel sluggish, losing those extra pounds could make a big difference. There are also other factors to consider. For example, if you are at risk of developing diabetes or heart disease, or have high cholesterol, shedding those extra pounds could make the difference between staying healthy or developing a chronic illness.

So how do you lose weight without gaining it back? Not by dieting. One of the problems is that we Americans are obsessed with dieting and, ironically, this very obsession may prevent us from maintaining a stable, normal weight. Practically every month a new "miracle" diet sweeps the nation, and millions of us slavishly follow it. Initially, most of these diets do work in that they help us to shed pounds, often very quickly. Nearly all of these fad diets, however, fall short in that they do not have a lasting effect, or more accurately, they are very difficult to follow for more than a few weeks at a time. In fact, some studies have shown that as many as 90 percent of all dieters regain the weight within a year of losing it and, sadly, many put on even more weight.

Clearly, dieting alone is not the answer and may cause even more problems in the long run. If you are obese or overweight enough that you should lose weight, in order to achieve your goal, you will need to take a multifaceted approach.

Concentrate on health—Throw out the scale, forget about losing weight, and focus on health. You want to feel strong, vital, and healthy, and that should be your motivation, not the short-term goal of losing a few pounds. Your permanent goal should be to achieve a healthy lifestyle.

Consume fewer calories—You will need to cut back on calories, but not necessarily on food. Eating fewer calories means filling up on high-fiber, low-calorie, nutrient-dense foods such as fruits, vegetables, and whole grains.

Foods that are high in fat are particularly bad, because each gram of fat contains nine calories versus four calories for each gram of protein or carbohydrate. This does not mean however, that fat-free foods can be eaten carte blanche. I believe that one of the primary reasons that Americans are getting fatter is due to the popular misconception that fat-free foods can be eaten with impunity. This is simply not true. Fat-free foods (especially snack foods like cookies and chips) are laden with calories and, if you eat more calories than you expend, you will gain weight. It doesn't matter if those added calories are fat, protein, or carbohydrate, they add up!

Eat when you are hungry—Do not allow yourself to get too hungry, you will be tempted to binge. Don't try to fight your hunger, or ignore hunger pains. Rather, reach for the right foods when you crave a snack. Good snack foods include air-popped popcorn without the butter or oil, fresh vegetables with a splash of raspberry vinegar or a low-fat yogurt dip.

Cut back naturally—Very often, the problem is that we reach for food even when we are not really hungry. I have developed a system that helps me know when to eat, and when to stop. I rely on my "hunger gauge." Here's what I mean. On a scale of 0 to 10, 0 stands for empty or very hungry, 7 stands for satiety, and 10 stands for overstuffed. Before I eat, I put my hand on my stomach and close my eyes. If I am only slightly hungry, I rate myself a 5, and I wait until I'm at 3 before I eat. When I eat, I stop eating by the time I'm at 6—I may not feel completely satisfied, but I am certainly no longer hungry. I never eat beyond 7. I have found that this simple program of self-regulation is all it takes to help people lose weight without dieting.

Increase your expenditure of energy—Calories are converted into energy, and energy is the fuel that keeps the body running. If energy is not used up by activity as nature intended, it is converted into fat, and that is what puts on those extra pounds. The human body works best when we are physically active, yet most of us live inactive, sedentary lives. Getting regular exercise is the most critical component of any exercise program. Walk briskly for at least one half-hour each day, jog, run, play tennis, do weight training, take an aerobics class, whatever you do, keep yourself on the go.

Water, water, and more water—Drink eight to ten glasses of water daily, and try to drink at least one of those glasses of water right before mealtime. It will give you a sensation of feeling full, and you will eat less, I guarantee it.

Spice up your act—Many people complain that foods that are low in fat tend to be bland and flavorless. Although it's true that fat does impart a bit of flavor to food, and certainly improves "mouth feel," there is no reason you must sacrifice taste when you are trying to eat light. You can more than compensate for any loss in flavor by adding herbs and spices to your food. Most Americans use only a handful of herbs and spices (salt and pepper are the most common) but foreign cuisines, which are literally packed with flavor and low in fat, rely heavily on natural seasonings. A sprinkle of cinnamon, a dash of curry powder, a pinch of caraway, sauteed garlic, diced onion, or a touch of cayenne can perk up the blandest dish. (By the way, all of these herbs are also natural remedies that can help prevent disease. For more information, I refer you to *Earl Mindell's Herb Bible.*)

Add fiber to your diet—Foods that are high in fiber will fill you up without filling you out. The National Cancer Institute recommends that Americans eat between 20 and 40 grams of fiber daily in the form of whole grains, fruits, and vegetables. Few Americans actually eat this much fiber. I think that if more did, there would be far fewer cases of obesity.

The real cure for obesity is the kinds of changes in diet and lifestyle that I have just outlined: There is no "magic bullet" when it comes to weight loss and, unfortunately, few supplements to recommend. These few supplements, however, may help.

Minerals

Chromium picolinate—Chromium picolinate (the most effective form of chromium) will not help you lose weight, but can help to increase muscle mass if you are already working out. In other words, chromium picolinate will help you build muscle mass, which will give you a sleeker, more attractive look.

Chromium can also help maintain a normal blood-sugar level; many people experience a dip in blood sugar during midmorning and midafternoon, and that is the time they may run for a quick (and fattening) snack. Chromium helps to stabilize blood-sugar levels, thus preventing the kinds of dips and spikes that could trigger binge eating. New research has shown that 1000 mcg. of chromium picolinate given

to adult onset diabetics has helped to lower their blood sugar. For .
ing weight, I recommend doses of 200–600 mcg. daily.

Personal Advice

Beware salad bars—Many people who are trying to lose weight mistakenly believe that any food that includes the word *salad* is low fat and low calorie. Nothing could be further from the truth. Salad bars can be laden with foods (such as egg salad and tuna salad) that are dripping with mayonnaise and fatty dressings. Here's my advice: Fill up your plate with fresh vegetables, then place a few tablespoons of your favorite salad dressing in a separate bowl. Dip your fork in the salad dressing before picking up each biteful of salad; the fork will be coated with just enough flavor to keep you happy, but you will be spared many of the calories and much of the fat.

Slow down—Your mother was right—eat more slowly! It takes the stomach twenty minutes to signal to your brain that you are full. If you eat quickly, you will overeat.

Don't eat while watching TV, while in a movie, or in a moving vehicle. This is called *unconscious eating*, and you will definitely overeat. Fast-food restaurants are a no-no. They make you eat *fast*, not to mention the fact that they offer high-fat, calorie-laden fare.

Earl's Rx

Multivitamin with minerals: If you are trying to lose weight, be sure to take a good multivitamin with minerals daily so that you are getting the necessary nutrients. If you are nutrient deprived, you will be hungry, tired, and more likely to overeat.

Chromium picolinate: One 200 mcg. tablet or capsule up to three times daily.

Osteoporosis

Osteoporosis afflicts some 24 million Americans.

One out of three women over age fifty will suffer vertebral fractures and hip fractures as a result of this disease.

Osteoporosis is not for women only: one out of six men will get this disease.

Osteoporosis is a degenerative bone disorder characterized by the thinning and weakening of bone, leaving it more vulnerable to breaks and fractures.

Your skeleton is a hotbed of activity. From childhood on through adulthood, old bone is continually being replaced with new bone in a process called *remodeling*. During remodeling, bone-eating cells called *osteoclasts* break down bone tissue creating microscopic cavities. Then bone-forming cells, called *osteoblasts,* refill the cavities with fresh tissue. During childhood and adolescence, bone-builders form more new tissue than bone-eaters take away. But some time, usually after age thirty, bone-eaters begin to outnumber bone-builders, setting the stage for osteoporosis.

Postmenopausal women are especially prone to osteoporosis, in fact, about half of them will develop this disease. This tendency should not be surprising, since estrogen is involved in the absorption of calcium by the bones, which is critical for the formation of new bone. As estrogen levels drop after menopause, every woman experiences an acceleration in the rate of bone loss. Small-boned, slender Caucasian and Asian women are at greatest risk of developing osteoporosis. Women who are heavy drinkers (more than two alcoholic beverages daily) and who smoke are also at a higher risk of becoming osteoporotic.

Although most people think of osteoporosis as a problem that strikes small-boned women, about 15 percent of all men will also suffer problems related to osteoporosis.

Studies have shown that most women underestimate the seriousness of osteoporosis; in fact, three out of four postmenopausal women have never discussed osteoporosis with their doctors. Women clearly do not view osteoporosis with the same urgency as they do cancer or even heart disease. This can be a serious mistake. About 40 percent of all postmenopausal women will develop vertebral fractures that can result in the rounded back or "dowager's hump." More than three hundred thousand postmenopausal women will get hip fractures, which not only will leave many women permanently disabled but can be deadly: about 20 percent of all women who fracture their hips die within six months of the injury due to complications such as pneumonia.

There is no easy answer to osteoporosis. Osteoporosis is a complex condition involving hormonal, lifestyle, nutritional, and environmental factors. There is no cure for this condition, but exercise, diet, supplements and, for women, hormone-replacement therapy can help stop further bone loss and in some instances may actually help strengthen bone density. For men, exercise and supplements may help to keep bones straight and strong.

Minerals

Calcium—Almost 100 percent of the body's calcium resides in teeth and bones, which makes calcium intake and absorption vital to bone health. Therefore, a diet rich in calcium, along with vitamin D, which helps the small intestine absorb calcium, is crucial to the prevention of osteo porosis. A 1990 study from Tufts University found that calcium supplements can slow bone loss in women who are more than five years past menopause and do not get enough calcium. (Postmenopausal women are advised to take between 1200 and 1500 mg. of calcium daily.)

Fluoride—Fluoride is a mineral that is essential in the formation of teeth and bone. It is available in seafood, gelatin, and in the drinking water of about 45 percent of all communities in the United States. There is no RDA (Recommended Daily Allowance), but the National Academy of Sciences estimates safe and adequate dietary intake is between 1.5 and 4 mg. Doses exceeding 20 mg. per day can produce toxic effects.

Researchers at the Southwestern Medical Center in Dallas studied about one hundred postmenopausal women. Half received 800 mg. of calcium citrate (a form of calcium believed to be well absorbed by the body), the other half received the same amount of calcium plus treatment with an experimental slow-release form of sodium fluoride. After two-and-a-half years, the mineral content of the spinal bones in the fluoride-calcium group had increased, while the group that received calcium only saw no change in bone-mineral content. Not only that, but the calcium only group suffered twice the number of new fractures as the fluoride group. The conclusion of the study was that a carefully balanced regimen of calcium and slow-release fluoride stimulates new bone growth in people with osteoporosis.

Special combinations of fluoride and calcium are available by prescription. Talk to your doctor for more information.

Magnesium—Magnesium is apparently as important as calcium in maintaining proper bone health, because it is essential for calcium and vitamin C metabolism. In a recent two-year study, a group of menopausal women were given magnesium hydroxide to assess the effects of magnesium on bone density. At the end of the study, magnesium appears to have prevented fractures and resulted in significant increase in bone density. (The RDA for adults is 250 to 350 mg. daily. Too much magnesium can cause diarrhea and impaired kidney function; do not exceed 1000 mg. daily.)

Good food sources of magnesium include bananas; apricots; curry powder; wheat bran; seed food including whole grains, nuts, and beans; seafood; apricots; dried mustard; curry powder; and dark leafy vegetables.

Boron—Another mineral, boron, works with calcium and magnesium to promote strong bones. USDA researchers tested the effect of boron deficiency on twelve postmenopausal women. For 119 days, women were given 2000-calorie diets which were very low in boron. The women were later given the same diet, this time supplemented with 3 mg. of boron a day for forty-eight days. Researchers found that the boron supplement reduced the loss of calcium and magnesium in the urine and also dramatically elevated blood levels of estrogen and calcium, all of which can help preserve precious bone. (Doses in excess of 10 mg. of boron a day are not recommended.)

Vitamins

Vitamin D—Calcium cannot be absorbed without the addition of vitamin D. Vitamin D is found in many dairy products and is also manufactured by skin exposed to ten to twenty minutes of sunlight per week. While too much vitamin D is harmful, supplements of 400 international units (IU) daily are considered safe.

Herbs

Horsetail—This herb helps the body absorb and utilize calcium.

Dong quai—Chinese women rely on an herb, dong quai, and sip ginseng tea, which is also high in phytoestrogens, to control the discomfort of menopause. Phytoestrogens are also believed to help prevent bone loss.

Other Supplements

Fish oil—Certain types of food, mostly fish, are rich in a type of polyunsaturated fat known as omega-3 fatty acids. In a recent study, omega-3 fatty acids were shown to reduce renal excretion of calcium, increase calcium absorption by the bone, and thwart the action of the bone-breaking osteoclasts while stimilating the action of the bone-builder osteoblast. Good food sources include white tuna, salmon, mackerel, herring, lake trout, cod, flounder, and halibut. Fish-oil supplements are also available.

Acidophilus—These friendly bacteria that live in the intestine synthesize vitamin K, which is essential for the formation of osteocalcin. Why is this important in regard to osteoporosis? Osteocalcin enables calcium to be crystallized and transported into the bones. A low level of osteocalcin is a risk factor for developing osteoporosis. Acidophilus is found in unpasteurized yogurt (which is also a terrific source of calcium) and is available in the form of crystals or powder which can be added to juice or food.

Proanthocyanidins and anthocyanidins—These types of flavonoids are responsible for the deep red-blue color of many berries including: hawthorn berries, blackberries, blueberries, cherries, and raspberries. They are remarkable in their ability to stabilize collagen structures.
Since bone consists of collagen, supplementation with concentrated extracts or high intake of berries rich in these flavonoids may offer significant benefit in preventing osteoporosis.

Bone up on soy—Soybeans and soy products such as tofu, miso, and soy-based soups are rich in phytoestrogens, a hormonelike substance that mimics estrogen in humans. Since bone cells have estrogen receptors, it is probable that the plant estrogens in soy may bind to these receptors and act like natural estrogen.

Personal Advice

Weight-bearing exercise such as walking, tennis, dancing, low-impact aerobics, and specific exercises to strengthen and support your back, are recommended. Overall, it is important to reduce the intake of substances known to contribute to calcium loss. Among these are caffeinated beverages, cola drinks containing phophates, alcohol, and salt.

Being overweight puts an added strain on thinning bones. The "weight creep" that is so typical of age is probably attributable to lower levels of physical activity. Therefore, even if caloric intake is not increased, it may be vital to increase your exercise level to maintain a constant weight.

Since bone fractures are more prevalent and cause more complications in people with osteoporosis it is advisable to avoid exercises where falls are common such as skating, biking on rough terrain, and skiing.

It is also important to protect magnesium stores by avoiding the magnesium wasters: saturated fats, soft drinks, and caffeine.

Dairy products are an excellent source of calcium but can be a high source of fat. Use low-fat or skim milk and low-fat dairy products.

Earl's Rx

Try these bone builders!

Complete multivitamin with full-spectrum antioxidants: There are many antioxidant vitamin and mineral formulas on the market. I recommend one that includes alpha- and betacarotene, vitamins C and E, and selenium.

Magnesium: Take 500 mg. daily.

Calcium and vitamin D: Postmenopausal women should take 1500 mg. of calcium daily with 400 IU vitamin D. Men over age 50 should take 1000 mg. of calcium daily with 400 IU of vitamin D.

Grapeseed extract and green-tea extract combination: Take two to three tablets daily.

Acidophilus: One tablespoon of acidophilus powder or one capsule one-half hour before each meal.

Pain

Pain is the symptom that drives more people to seek medical attention than any other.

Billions of dollars are spent on medication to alleviate pain in the United States every day.

I magine if you lost the ability to feel pain. You might not know when you stepped on a nail, when you burned you hand, or that you were suffering from a potentially dangerous illness. Pain is an immediate response to injury, serving as nature's warning that something is wrong. Few of us think of pain as a good thing, yet clearly pain serves a very important purpose. If pain is not too severe and only temporary, it is not a real problem. Pain can become a real problem, however, if it is severe, chronic, and interferes with our ability to lead a full and active life.

Pain sensation is transmitted to the brain via sense receptors of the nervous system known as *nociceptors,* which are located throughout the body. When these sense organs are stimulated either by injury or stress, they convert that stimulation into impulses that are transmitted along certain peripheral nerve fibers to the spinal cord, and ultimately to the brain.

Opiate drugs, such as morphine, and certain naturally occurring substances produced within the brain, can inhibit the transmission of pain impulses or can block the nerve impulses that give rise to pain before they have a chance to reach the brain.

Drugs like morphine act on opiate receptors to make use of the naturally occurring opiates, called *endorphins,* that the body produces to block pain transmission. The problem is that continued use gradually depletes the effectiveness of the drug, demanding an ever-increasing dose to initiate pain relief and can become addictive. To make matters worse, over time painkillers can become ineffective, but the pain will still persist.

Chronic pain presents an even greater challenge to physicians and natural healers. Researchers believe that in chronic pain the input of pain messages via the nociceptor neurons play less of a role and that more activity seems to be generated in the central nervous system itself. The theory is that chronic pain persists because the pain signals are stimulated in much the same way that memory is stored, eventually making cells hyperexcitable to a familiar sensation. In other words, cells remember the sensation, and the slightest stimulation starts the process going.

Scientists are developing new compounds to target chronic pain that doesn't really respond to current pain-altering medicines. There are several new drugs on the drawing board, and for people with constant, unrelenting pain, these new treatments may be true lifesavers. For the usual aches and pains that affect most people, however, natural remedies may do the trick.

Vitamins

Choline and B complex—Choline and B-complex (B1, B2, B6) provide the raw material needed to produce endorphins, the body's natural painkillers. B complex also helps us cope with stress and, as anyone who has ever experienced chronic pain knows, it can be very stressful. The B vitamins are most plentiful in unrefined whole grains such as wheat, rice, oats, and rye, green leafy vegetables, meats, poultry, fish, eggs, nuts, beans, liver, and brewer's yeast.

Minerals

Copper, calcium, and manganese—Our diets—or, more particularly, the amount of minerals in our diets—may play a role in general aches and pains not related to an injury, infection, or chronic illness. One fascinating study sponsored by the USDA at the Human Nutrition Research Center analyzed patient records from eight separate nutrition studies for medications dispensed for nonspecific pain by researchers. In each of the studies, patients lived at the facilities where the studies were being done. In the subjects whose diets were the most severely restricted, pain medication was requested three times more frequently than those who ate more well-rounded meals.

Men and women with a lower-than-normal intake of copper had a much higher rate of pain-killer use than those who consumed normal amounts of copper. In addition, researchers found that young women took more pain medication when their diets were low in both calcium and manganese. Finally, and perhaps not surprisingly, the researchers noted that obese young women who were participating in a weight-loss study requested pain medication more often when their caloric intake was cut in half. In this case, psychological factors, such as a feeling of deprivation, may increase the need for painkillers.

Herbs

Capsaicin—For centuries, herbalists have recommended applying a paste made with chili peppers to the skin to treat muscle and joint pains. They knew that the paste would initially sting but, once the stinging stopped, the pain would miraculously disappear, often for hours on end. These early healers did not know how this paste worked its magic. Today we know that capsaicin, the compound in chili peppers that gives them their hot, stinging taste is the same substance that relieves pain when applied directly to skin. When rubbed on skin, capsaicin cream stimulates the production of substance P, a chemical in the nerve cells of the skin that sends the pain message to the brain. Capsaicin quickly depletes the cells of substance P and once it is used up, the brain no longer knows that it is supposed to feel pain and, so, we don't. Several topical preparations containing capsaicin are available over-the-counter and are growing in popularity. Aerosol sprays containing capsaicin are also used to treat cluster headaches. (See "Headache," p. 132.)

Meadowsweet—In 1853, German scientists used extracts from the herb meadowsweet to concoct the most famous pain reliever of all time—aspirin. In fact, the word *aspirin* was derived from *acetylsalicylic acid,* a compound in meadowsweet, and from the Latin word for meadowsweet, *spiraea.* Meadowsweet by itself is low in salicylate, a major component of aspirin, but it is less likely to cause aspirin's major side effect, stomach upset. It is excellent for nonspecific aches and pains.

White willow—This herb contains more salicylate than aspirin, and it is recommended for headache, fever, arthritis, inflammation, and other pain.

Other Supplements

D,L phenylalanine—This amino acid can enhance the action of naturally produced endorphins or painkillers, thus reducing the need for painkillers in some people. Some studies have shown D,L phenylalanine to be very helpful in terms of controlling pain, while others have shown it to have little, if any, effect. My advice is to try it and see if it can work for you in combination with other herbal remedies such as white willow.

Personal Advice

First, remember pain is an exquisitely designed warning system to let us know when we are in trouble. If you suffer from pain, see your physician or natural healer to find out the cause.

Other noninvasive methods of treating pain include biofeedback, acupuncture, and meditation. Nonstressful exercise such as yoga, tai chi, and swimming can help control pain especially for pain associated with arthritis, backache, and other chronic conditions.

Earl's Rx

B complex: One 50 mg. tablet with meals up to three times daily.

Calcium and magnesium: Take 500 mg. calcium and 250 mg. magnesium three times daily, one-half hour after meals.

d l phenylalanine: One or two tablets or capsules every three to four hours for pain, between meals.

White willow bark: One or two capsules every three to four hours for pain.

Feverfew: 500 mg. capsules, one to three daily.

Pregnancy

A common B vitamin (folic acid) can protect against serious forms of birth defects.

The question every mother-to-be asks is, "What can I do to have a healthy baby?" There are a few basic things you should know.

During pregnancy, it is simply not possible to get enough vitamins and minerals to sustain your needs and those of your developing baby's by food alone. Therefore, your doctor or natural healer should prescribe a supplement of essential vitamins and minerals. (Since anything you eat or drink can cross the placenta, please do not take any medication or supplements unless it is under the supervision of your doctor or natural healer.)

Vitamins

Folic acid—Don't underestimate the importance of getting the right amount of vitamins. In fact, a recent study showed that one single B vitamin, folic acid, can virtually wipe out one of the most common forms of birth defects. A study reported in *The Lancet* (1994), concluded that folic-acid supplements (400 mcg. daily) can significantly reduce the incidence of neural-tube defects including spina-bifida, a serious and life-threatening deformity of the spinal column.

Folic acid may also protect against facial deformities. Researchers from the California Birth Defects Monitoring Program found that taking folic acid prior to becoming pregnant and during the first two months of pregnancy may reduce the incidence of cleft lip (known as harelip) and cleft palate. The California team surveyed 731 women whose children had these deformities and 734 women whose children had no birth defects. Women who had taken multivitamins, which ordinarily contain folic acid, had fewer children with oral or facial deformities. In fact, researchers found that taking multivitamins reduced the risk of these conditions by 25 to 50 percent.

Excellent sources of folic acid include brussels sprouts, cauliflower, broccoli, oranges, orange juice, bananas, liver, eggs, whole-meal bread and fortified cereal. Folic-acid supplements should be taken up to and during the first twelve weeks of pregnancy. The usual recommendation for pregnant women is 400 mcg. daily.

Antioxidants—A pregnant woman's diet should be rich in antioxidants such as betacarotene, vitamins C and E, and selenium, and these important vitamins and minerals should be included in her prenatal vitamin regimen. Here's why. A recent study done at the University of Cincinnati showed that women with preeclampsia (a dangerous form of high blood pressure that strikes during pregnancy) had only half as much antioxidant activity in their blood as women who do not get this disorder. This doesn't mean that antioxidants can prevent preeclampsia, but it clearly suggests that they have a role to play in keeping women healthy during pregnancy.

Another recent study reported indicates a mother-to-be may be able to help prevent a future brain tumor in her unborn child. New research strongly suggests that a mother's diet just before and in the first few weeks of pregnancy may influence later development of one of the most common types of childhood brain tumors. In particular, a maternal diet low in Vitamin C may make contribute to the formation of brain tumors in small children.

Vitamin A—Pregnant women should not take vitamin A in large doses (over 5000 IU daily) since it has been linked to birth defects. It is far preferable to stick to betacarotene, which is converted to vitamin A as the body needs it, therefore, there is little chance of overdosing on vitamin A.

Minerals

Magnesium—Can magnesium help prevent preeclampsia? A study evaluated blood magnesium levels in twenty-seven patients with preeclampsia and twenty-seven healthy pregnant women. Magnesium levels before treatment with magnesium were significantly lower in the women with preeclampsia than in the healthy controls. This study suggests that low magnesium concentrations may contribute to the development of hypertension. Many nutritionally oriented doctors today recommend magnesium supplements for their patients who are prone to develop preeclampsia.

Zinc—Low zinc intake during pregnancy may be associated with an increased risk of low birth weight and preterm delivery. In one study, zinc consumption was assessed by asking women to recall their dietary intake. Women who consumed 40 percent of the RDA for zinc during pregnancy doubled the risk of having a low birth weight or preterm infant compared to those with moderate zinc intake. There was more than a threefold increased risk for preterm delivery. Another study evaluated 580 healthy African-American pregnant women with plasma zinc levels below normal. The women were divided into groups. One group received zinc supplementation, the other was given a placebo. Infants of women taking the zinc supplement group had a significantly greater birth weight and head circumference, a sign of general health.

Calcium—Calcium supplements can reduce blood pressure during pregnancy, which can help to protect against preeclampsia. In one study of nearly 1200 women, starting in their twentieth week of pregnancy, one group received 2 grams per day of calcium carbonate or a placebo. All women were followed to the end of their pregnancies. At the end of the study, the rates of high blood pressure or related problems were lower in the calcium-taking group than in the placebo group.

These findings are consistent with other studies of women in countries such as Guatemala and Ethiopia, where the typical diet is low in calories but high in calcium. In these countries, although these women are not eating as well as American women, they still have a lower incidence of high blood pressure during pregnancy and related problems, such water retention and *proteinuria* (the presence of protein in the urine that might indicate kidney disease caused by high blood pressure).

Yet another study of American women confirms that calcium can help reduce high blood pressure during pregnancy. Researchers gave thirty women with normal blood pressure and twenty women with elevated blood pressure a 1000 mg. per day calcium supplement over a twenty-week period. Women with high blood pressure experienced a dramatic drop in diastolic pressure, (the pressure in the arteries when the heart muscle relaxes between beats), but no change in systolic pressure. Calcium did not appear to have any affect on women with normal blood pressure.

Iron—A report in *American Journal of Clinical Nutrition* notes that maternal iron deficiency diagnosed at the onset of pregnancy was associated with low energy, inadequate weight gain, and a twofold or greater increase in the risks of preterm delivery and low birth weight. The moral is that during pregnancy it is essential to eat foods that are rich in iron. In many cases, physicians or natural healers will prescribe iron supplements to their pregnant patients.

Herbs

Raspberry leaf This is the most widely used and safest herb to prepare the uterus for delivery since it is virtually nontoxic even at high doses. Drink one cup of raspberry tea daily.

Ginger—This root has been used by Chinese healers for centuries as an antinausea measure for motion sickness, morning sickness during pregnancy, and general stomach upset. It is considered safe for pregnant women. To alleviate nausea and discomfort caused by hormonal changes, drink a cup of ginger-root tea or take a ginger-root tablet or capsule first thing in the morning. Throughout the day, sip ginger ale or peppermint tea.

Chamomile—This tea is a great stress reliever and combined with ginger is recommended for morning sickness.

Dandelion greens and roots—This plant has a high percentage of quality betacarotene, calcium, and iron. They also have a gentle diuretic action that helps rid the body of excess water but because the leaf is high in natural potassium, it does not deplete potassium in the system as do synthetic diuretics.

Centella—This herb has been used in Asian medicine for hundreds of years for the treatment of skin sores and infections. It has been found to be most helpful in helping to heal an episiotomy (the incision of the vulva sometimes performed during the second stage of delivery to avoid tearing). Women who take centella report less pain and more rapid healing than women subjected to standard measures. Many women also find that centella is useful to help treat varicose veins that may develop after pregnancy. (Centella should not be used during pregnancy.)

Butchers broom—Hours of labor can result in nasty hemorrhoids. For relief, try applying a salve made from this herb.

Other Supplements

Omega-3 fatty acids—Omega-3 fatty acids have been used in high-risk pregnancies to prevent miscarriage; researchers believe that they may prevent the formation of blood clots in the placenta, and also help to keep maternal blood pressure within normal levels. Omega-3 fatty acids are found in fish, flaxseed, or a fish-oil supplement. If you have a history of miscarriage, you should talk to your doctor about taking omega-3 fatty acids.

Personal Advice

Eating for two—The nutritional demands of pregnancy are extraordinary both for healthy development of the baby and to maintain the health of the mother. Remember, a developing baby will get the nutrients it needs for growth at the mother's expense, if necessary.

Protein needs during pregnancy increase also. However, in the United States women can get the needed protein from milk, meat, fish, tofu, poultry, or cheese, without drastically changing their diets.

Since constipation is a common problem in pregnancy, getting enough fiber from bran, fruits, prunes, and raw vegetables is important. Proper diet, along with enough fluids, daily exercise, a stress-free environment, and sufficient sleep will all help to achieve a successful pregnancy and delivery. Hemorrhoids are one of the more unpleasant effects pregnancy has on the body. Diet can go a long way in controlling this condition. Unprocessed bran, lots of fruits, vegetables, and whole grains will add fiber to the diet and drinking lots of water will help soften the stool.

Weight gain is important to nourish the fetus, but obesity increases the changes of complications, and should be considered before a woman becomes pregnant.

If heartburn is a problem, eat small more frequent meals rather than three large meals a day. Mint tea can help relieve the gassy feeling.

What to avoid—What is not good for you is not good for the baby. The list of things to avoid includes alcohol, tobacco, caffeine, and illegal drugs (and sometimes even over-the-counter drugs unless prescribed by your doctor).

Alcohol is one drug that should be avoided by all pregnant woman.

Because the first two months after conception are so critical, and since optimal amounts of alcohol have not been determined, anyone planning a pregnancy should stop drinking before attempting conception. Drinking alcohol during pregnancy can cause fetal alcohol syndrome, which can result in mental retardation; brain, heart, and nervous system problems; and facial abnormalities.

Smoking is another habit that should be eliminated before conceiving. Smoking can cause problems before, during, and after your pregnancy. Some studies show that smokers may have more difficulty becoming pregnant, and others show that it can increase the chance of first trimester miscarriage, and/or premature labor. Smoking can also have long-lasting detrimental effects on your child. A study reported in *Pediatrics* evaluated four hundred families. Children in the group whose mothers smoked ten or more cigarettes per day during pregnancy had a lower intelligence score that those whose mothers did not smoke during pregnancy. The conclusion: Smoking during pregnancy appears to result in neurodevelopmental impairment.

It isn't only women who affect their babies by smoking. The number of sperm and the percentage of motile sperm decrease significantly in smokers, according to how much the man smokes and the duration of his smoking habit. Paternal smoking, in particular, appears to increase the risk of birth defects and childhood cancer in offspring. Conclusion: Paternal smoking appears to result in damage not only to their own DNA but also to the DNA of their sperm, an effect that may reverberate down future generations.

I advise women to avoid caffeine during pregnancy. Some studies suggest that caffeine intake before and during pregnancy may be associated with an increased risk of miscarriage.

Illegal drug use should stop before you conceive, and most certainly the moment the pregnancy begins. Even some over-the-counter drugs can affect a developing baby, so it is very important to tell your doctor about every medicine you are taking. Some drugs can damage a fetus in the first few weeks before the pregnancy is confirmed, so anyone planning a pregnancy should discuss this issue with a physician even before conception occurs.

Avoid exposure to poisons at work or at home. That includes x-rays, some cleaning products, lead, and chemicals.

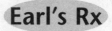

Earl's Rx

Your doctor or natural healer will prescribe a prenatal multivitamin that should include most everything that you need, therefore I am not going to suggest that you take a lot of extra supplements. Be sure, however, that your multivitamin contains at least 400 mcg. of folic acid and vitamins C, E, selenium, calcium, and zinc.

If you are prone to high blood pressure, ask your doctor about prescribing extra calcium and magnesium.

For morning sickness: Take two ginger capsules upon waking. Drink one cup of peppermint tea.

To prepare for labor: Drink one cup of raspberry tea daily.

Premenstrual Syndrome (PMS)

About 50 percent of menstruating women suffer from some form of premenstrual syndrome.

Symptoms range from mild to debilitating.

Diet, vitamin and mineral supplements, and in some cases, hormone therapy, can help reduce symptoms.

P remenstrual syndrome (PMS) is a common problem associated with symptoms such as headache, irritability, bloating, and insomnia prior to menstruation.

Although the term *premenstrual syndrome* was coined in 1931, when researchers first suggested that the condition was due to a hormonal imbalance related to the menstrual cycle, until recently many doctors didn't take women's complaints seriously. It was commonly believed that these types of problems were psychological rather than physical. Today we know better.

It has now been determined that the causes of PMS involve an imbalance of estrogen, prolactin, adrenal, and thyroid hormones. These fluctuating levels of hormones can effect mood, behavior, and physical changes.

This doesn't mean that natural changes that occur in women's bodies during menstruation should be treated as an illness; PMS is best viewed as a collection of symptoms that can be relieved through diet, exercise, nutritional supplements, herbs and, in severe cases, hormone therapy.

Both physical and emotional factors affect hormonal regulation, therefore, you not only have to learn how to improve your diet but how to deal with stress and emotional problems.

Diet

Even before you consider using supplements for PMS, be sure that you are eating the right foods. Eat a well-balanced, low-fat diet with adequate amounts of protein, fiber, and complex carbohydrates. Cut out excess salt, sugar, caffeine, and alcohol. Studies have shown that compared to

229

women who don't experience premenstrual distress, PMS patients consume almost twice as much carbohydrates, dairy products, and sodium; considerably more refined sugar; and less iron, manganese, and zinc. In addition, PMS patients showed lower levels of thiamine, riboflavin, and vitamin B6, a sign that these women should be eating more whole grains and less refined bleached-out bread and cake products.

Minerals

Zinc—At the Baylor College of Medicine in Texas, researchers tested zinc levels of both women with premenstrual syndrome symptoms and those without, and determined that some of the women with PMS had lower zinc levels during the ovulation phase of their monthly cycles. A deficiency in zinc may lead to a decreased secretion of progesterone, endorphins and other natural opiates, which in turn can aggravate the symptoms of PMS.

Magnesium—Magnesium deficiency is strongly implicated as a possible cause of PMS. In a report published in *The Journal of the American College of Nutrition* researchers determined a magnesium deficiency has been associated with premenstrual syndrome alone or in combination with inadequacies of zinc, linoleic acid and B vitamins (predominantly B6).

PMS patients given a multivitamin and mineral supplement containing high doses of magnesium and vitamin B6, showed a 70 percent improvement of symptoms.

Vitamins

Vitamin A—High doses of vitamin A in the second half of the menstrual cycle have been shown to relieve symptoms. However, betacarotene is a better choice, since it is less toxic and is converted into vitamin A as the body needs it. Good food sources of betacarotene include apricots, sweet potatoes, broccoli, cantaloupe, pumpkin, carrots, mangoes, peaches, and spinach. Betacarotene is included in most antioxidant formulas, and is also available as a single supplement.

Vitamin E—Vitamin E supplements have been shown to reduce symptoms of tension, headache, fatigue, depression, and insomnia associated with PMS.

Vitamin B6—B6 is a natural diuretic and helps to relieve bloating and other symptoms of PMS. Combined with other B vitamins, it is also a wonderful stress reliever.

Herbs

Gingko biloba—A time-honored herbal remedy may be effective in treating a problem of modern women. A recent double-blind study to determine ginkgo biloba's effectiveness in treating PMS studied 165 women between the ages of eighteen and forty-five who suffered from such symptoms as bloating and breast tenderness before the onset of menstruation. The women were either given a placebo or treated with ginkgo extract from day sixteen of one menstrual period to day five of the next. Test results showed that the ginkgo extract was effective in relieving many of the symptoms associated with PMS.

Licorice—The medicinal use of licorice root was known to herbal healers for thousands of years. Today scientists have determined that an increase in the estrogen-to-progesterone ratio accounts for many of the symptoms of PMS. The major active component of licorice root is *glycyrrhizin* (also known as *glycyrrhizic acid* or *glycyrrhizinic acid*), a compound that is believed to help normalize estrogen levels. Licorice is included in many herbal preparations designed for women. Caution: Licorice can cause a rise in blood pressure and should not be used by women who have been diagnosed with high blood pressure, or who have borderline high blood pressure.

Dong quai—Dong quai has been called nature's gift to women. It is an all-purpose herb grown in China, where it has traditionally been used for a wide range of female complaints. It is a tonic for the female reproductive system, and helps regulate the menstrual cycle, especially the imbalances which are responsible for some of the symptoms of premenstrual syndrome. Dong quai is rich in vitamins and minerals, including A, B12, and E.

Evening primrose—Evening primrose is an American herb that has been used by Native Americans for centuries. The oil from this plant is high in gamma linolenic acid, an essential polyunsaturated fatty acid that is converted into prostaglandin, a hormone necessary for many important body functions. Studies show it is effective in treating symptoms of PMS such as irritability, headaches, breast tenderness, and bloating.

Dandelion greens—These nutritious weeds are high in potassium and, unlike synthetic diuretics, they won't cause a deficiency of that essential mineral. Dandelion tea can help restore the body's proper water balance.

Vitex—Also called *chaste tree* or *chasteberry*, this herb is reputed to be a hormone regulator and is used to treat PMS. Studies suggest that it may increase the production of progesterone, which could help normalize the hormonal imbalance that is believed to cause PMS.

Wild yam—Wild yam contains natural progesterone, which may help PMS symptoms by restoring the estrogen/progesterone balance. Wild yam is available as a cream. It can be applied to thin skin such as the inside of the arms or legs, the face and neck, upper chest, and the abdomen. Be sure to follow instructions. According to John Lee, M.D., a well-known proponent of progesterone therapy, progesterone should only be used from days twelve through twenty-six of the menstrual cycle—if you use it other times, it could throw your cycle off. In addition, this product should not be used by someone being treated with prescribed estrogen or progesterone therapies. I recommend that women who want to use this natural hormonal therapy should do so under the supervision of a natural healer.

Personal Advice

A diet high in complex carbohydrates, which are found in vegetables, whole grains, beans and fruit; and low in fat, salt, sugar and alcohol, all four of which can cause water retention should help. Drinking six to eight glasses of water daily will help eliminate excess fluids. Natural diuretics such as watermelon, asparagus, and parsley will also help get rid of excess water.

Increase your intake of antioxidants (foods rich in vitamins C and E and selenium.) Fluctuating levels of sugar, and the body's subsequent interruption in its ability to handle insulin, can lead to a craving for sweets during the premenstrual phase. Eating smaller, more frequent meals will help stabilize blood-sugar levels. Eating sugary foods often initiates a vicious cycle of additional sugar cravings, as an increase in your body's need for B-complex vitamins creates craving for even more sugar.

Nicotine is a brain stimulant much like caffeine, and since stimulating the brain magnifies PMS symptoms, eliminating smoking and cutting back on coffee, tea, and cocoa is a good idea. PMS is often associated with disruptions in the normal sleep pattern. In addition to eliminating caffeine, a supplemental dose of melatonin might be helpful. (See "Sleep Disorders," p. 242.)

A nightcap is the worst thing you can do to promote sleep! Although alcohol initially makes you drowsy, it can cause frequent night awakenings. Alcohol also depletes the body of the B vitamins, disrupts the metabolism of carbohydrates, and affects the liver's ability to process hormones.

Exercise not only helps relieve stress, it can elevate your mood, strengthen your muscles, and improve alertness. Severe cases of PMS might benefit from hormone therapy. Consult your physician or natural healer; an endocrinologist can evaluate your body's hormonal balance. Nontraditional approaches to PMS include acupuncture, chiropractic adjustment, and therapeutic massage.

Earl's Rx

If you have PMS, I recommend the following.

Antioxidant formula: Any woman with PMS should take a good antioxidant combination daily that includes vitamin E and betacarotene. Take two capsules daily.

Vitamin B6: One 50–100 mg. tablet daily for ten days up to the onset of menstruation. You can stop when menstruation begins.

Evening primrose oil: One 500 mg. capsule up to three times daily for seven to ten days before onset of menstruation. You can stop when menstruation begins.

Ginkgo biloba: One 60 mg. capsule or tablet up to two times daily.

Vitex: One capsule, up to three times daily, beginning ten days before onset of menstruation. You can stop when menstruation begins.

Zinc: One 15 mg. capsule or tablet daily.

Magnesium: One 500 mg. capsule or tablet daily.

Prostate Gland Enlargement

Ten million American men suffer from benign prostatic hypertrophy (enlarged prostate gland) in the United States.

Herbs may offer an effective alternative to surgery.

The prostate is a small walnut-shaped gland that surrounds the part of the urethra that is located just below the bladder. As men age, the prostate gland has a tendency to enlarge or swell, obstructing the urethra, which can interfere with urination. The residual urine causes unpleasant symptoms, including a constant urge to urinate, burning, and even pain. The medical term for this condition is benign prostatic hypertrophy (BPH) and it is not in any way related to cancer of the prostate. (See page 66.) Nevertheless, the symptoms for both problems can be similar, and men who have experienced any of them should be seen by their physicians or natural healers for an accurate diagnosis. Most important, there is no reason for men to suffer in silence; there are many effective treatments that can virtually eliminate any discomfort that may be caused by an enlarged prostate.

Recently, natural remedies have also been proven to be as effective as some of the commonly used drugs.

Herbs

Saw palmetto berry—Long known to southeastern Native Americans, this herb acts directly on the enlarged prostate to reduce inflammation and pain, and also helps the bladder to empty efficiently. Double-blind studies by French and Italian researchers have shown that saw-palmetto supplements reduced the number of times men had to get up at night to urinate by nearly half, increased their flow rate of urine, and lessened residual urine by 42 percent.

Researchers believe that saw palmetto works by deactivating an enzyme (5 alpha reductase) that triggers the production of a more potent form of testosterone called *dihydrotestosterone,* which stimulates prostatic cell growth. In addition, saw palmetto is a mild anti-inflammatory. Saw palmetto is available in capsule form.

Pumpkin-seed oil—The seed from the pumpkin plant was known to Native Americans for its diuretic quality, and was used to ease the symptoms of enlarged prostate long before the settlers adopted it for the same purpose. There are many anecdotal reports of pumpkin seed helping to reduce symptoms in men with enlarged prostates. Pumpkin seeds are an excellent source of zinc, the mineral that is found in great abundance in the prostate.

Pygeum—Pygeum is a large evergreen tree, the bark of which is used for healing. Pygeum contains a natural anti-inflammatory which blocks the production of *prostaglandins,* hormonelike compounds that are involved in the inflammatory process.

Buchu leaf—This herb which is included in many herbal formulas for prostate health is a mild disinfectant that can help to prevent urinary tract infections and inflammation. It is also a mild diuretic that can stimulate urination.

Minerals

Zinc—For more than a decade, I have been recommending this mineral to all men for good prostate health. There are high levels of zinc found in the prostate gland and, clearly, this mineral is important for the proper maintenance of the male reproductive system. Zinc is also a well-known immune booster, and can thus also be useful in terms of preventing urinary-tract infections, which can irritate the prostate.

Personal Advice

Water—Drink lots of water; it will flush out bacteria that can cause urinary tract infections, which can aggravate the prostate.

Sitz bath—A warm bath can help to soothe an irritated prostate by reducing inflammation.

Lose weight—Researchers believe men who are overweight have a significantly higher incidence of enlarged prostate. Eat a low-fat diet that includes plenty of fruits and vegetables, grains, and legumes.

Earl's Rx

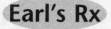

I recommend that you find a special combination formula that contains the following: Saw palmetto extract (150 mg.), pygeum africanum extract (50 mg.), and vitamin C for antixodant protection (I recommend calcium ascorbate because it is a more easily absorbed form.) Take two capsules daily with meals.

In addition, take the following:

Zinc: One 15–50 mg. capsule or tablet daily.

Psoriasis and Eczema

Approximately 4 million Americans suffer from psoriasis.

More than $1.5 billion is spent on prescription and over-the-counter drugs each year.

New therapies are now available to help control the disorders.

P soriasis and eczema are two common skin disorders that are both characterized by red, dry patchy, scaling skin. They are dissimilar in that psoriasis is caused by abnormal cell growth, and eczema is often caused by an allergy or skin irritation. In addition, psoriasis is closely linked to arthritis; in fact, 10 percent of all people with psoriasis develop arthritis or gout. Both psoriasis and eczema can be hereditary. Despite their differences, the treatment for both of these skin disorders is similar, at least for mild cases.

In biblical times, psoriasis sufferers were often banished to leper colonies. Thousands of years later, when introducing a new psoriasis lotion to the millions of Americans who suffer from the skin condition, Madison Avenue dubbed psoriasis "the heartbreak disease." The name stuck, and with good reason, as those who suffer from it know.

Psoriasis is a chronic disorder that causes scaly, red lesions on the skin. The lesions are caused by the excessive growth and shedding of skin cells. Normally, skin cells mature in about thirty days and are then shed from the body. In psoriasis, however, cells mature in only four days; the cause of this abnormal cell growth remains a mystery, although it is suspected there may be a genetic predisposition to this disease.

Although it is not contagious, it is often unsightly and embarrassing, causing others to be afraid of making close physical contact with the person suffering from the disorder. To add to the heartbreak, until quite recently, doctors could offer little hope for treating or curing the disease. It's more than embarrassment, however, that causes heartbreak. Depending on the severity and location of the lesions, it can also be very painful and at times itchy. In rare cases, certain forms of psoriasis may be life-threatening.

Although eczema is not life-threatening, it can cause great discomfort. Fortunately, there is now hope for both psoriasis and eczema patients. Although a cure is still elusive, many new medications, dietary changes, and other therapies are being used successfully to bring patients into remission.

Hydrocortisone creams are routinely used to treat both eczema and psoriasis and usually relieve symptoms quickly. Low-dose creams are sold over-the-counter while the more potent and effective creams are available only by prescription. The problem with hydrocortisone creams, however, is that they cannot be used for more than a few weeks at a time or they can cause the skin to thin. In addition, if they are overused, they can become ineffective.

Keeping skin well-moisturized is one way to help prevent an attack of eczema. There are many excellent over-the-counter moisture creams available, and even some stronger prescription moisture creams that work well. The trick is to moisturize your skin daily, even if you think you don't have to. Skin that is well-hydrated will be less likely to become irritated.

If you suffer from psoriasis, you may need to make changes in your lifestyle. For example, we know that the consumption of red meat, high-fat foods, yeast infections, and excessive alcohol intake can trigger psoriasis. So can stress, throat infections, and drugs such as lithium and quinidine. We also know that certain factors can help improve psoriasis, such as exposure to sunlight, keeping the skin well-moisturized, and even certain vitamins.

These supplements can help people with both psoriasis and eczema.

Vitamins

Vitamin D—The sunshine vitamin has been proven valuable in the treatment of psoriasis, and I suspect that it will also help eczema. An article in *Nutrition Review* (May 1992), reports that the body produces its own vitamin D when the skin is exposed to sunlight, but psoriasis and eczema patients miss out on this benefit because they are the very people who will most likely cover up their bodies when they are outdoors. In addition, many sunscreens block vitamin D. Supplemental vitamin D, in either pill or cream form, can offer an alternative. Because of possible toxic effects do not take more than 400 IU daily without a physician's supervision. Stronger forms of vitamin D are available by prescription for patients with severe psoriasis.

Vitamin A—The vitamin known as the skin vitamin has been used to treat skin problems such as psoriasis and acne. In fact, a potent synthetic form of vitamin A is available by prescription and may be used in severe cases of psoriasis. High doses of vitamin A can be dangerous, so if you are prone to psoriasis, or are experiencing an outbreak, I recommend increasing your intake of betacarotene, which is converted into vitamin A as the body needs it and is nontoxic. Some patients apply vitamin A oil from capsules directly on the skin lesions, and there is no harm in doing this, but it may not be as effective as taking it internally. *Oral retinoids* (synthetic versions of vitamin A) include etretinate and isotretinoin (trade names are Tegison and Accutane). Both have been effective in clearing extensive psoriatic lesions. Exactly how the retinoids work is not well understood, but it is known that retinoids are important in normalizing skin cells and decreasing the rate of proliferation. Its most serious side effect is the risk of birth defects, and is therefore not recommended for pregnant women.

Omega 3 fatty acids—A recent German study highlighted the anti-inflammatory benefits of *omega-3 fatty acids.* These oils quickly reduced inflammation in twenty patients suffering from psoriasis. Omega-3 fatty acids offer yet another benefit to psoriasis sufferers. Ten percent of psoriasis patients also develop a form of arthritis known as *psoriatic arthritis.* Studies show that 1 to 3 grams daily of omega-3 fish oils can help both conditions. Although studies have not been done on eczema patients, omega-3 fatty acids should also help reduce their skin inflammation.

Herbs

Gotu kola—This herb has long been used to soothe skin problems, including leprosy, in India, Malaysia, and parts of Eastern Europe. Modern homeopathic physicians use it for psoriasis, eczema, blisters, and other skin disorders.

One interesting, albeit small, study showed that a gotu kola cream can help relieve the painful scaly red welts of psoriasis. Out of the seven psoriasis sufferers who used the cream, five showed improvement within two months, and only one of the five experienced any recurrence within four months after the treatment ended. Gotu kola cream is not available commercially, but it is available in liquid extract, and there is no harm in simply rubbing it directly on a psoriasis lesion to see if it will help.

Aloe vera—This herb is one of the world's best moisturizers, and keeping the skin moist is the number-one priority for both psoriasis and eczema sufferers. Psoriasis lesions and eczema tend to be dry and flaky, and if they are not moisturized, they can become inflamed and even bleed. This is especially true in the winter months when dry heat and lack of sunshine can trigger outbreaks in many people who are prone to psoriasis. A dry environment can also create the kind of skin irritation that leads to eczema, so it is essential to keep the skin moist and supple.

Capsaicin—Capsaicin is the substance which gives the fiery bite to hot chili peppers, but it can also relieve pain. In fact, capsaicin cream is now widely recommended for people with arthritis; it now appears that it can also be useful for those who suffer from psoriasis. Researchers at the General Infirmary in Leeds, England, conducted a double-blind study on ten patients with severe psoriasis for eight weeks. Researchers applied 0.025 percent capsaicin cream to some of the patients' lesions four times daily. After six weeks, seven out of ten patients who received the capsaicin showed marked improvement, and even those who did not show any obvious improvement said that the treatment had relieved their itching. (Capsaicin may be too irritating for those with eczema.)

Yellow dock—This herb has been used to treat skin problems since the Middle Ages, and is included in many herbal formulas designed to treat skin problems, including psoriasis and eczema.

Minerals

Selenium—Found in onion, garlic, and broccoli, this mineral may help against the flaky dandruff so prevalent in psoriasis sufferers. Selenium is also available in supplement form.

Personal Advice

Let's talk turkey—A recent study reports that people suffering from psoriasis can find relief by including more turkey in their diet. Researchers are not sure whether the turkey itself helps, or whether psoriasis victims may benefit from eating a low-fat diet, since red meat is not recommended for those with this condition.

Normalize your weight—A sudden weight gain or loss may trigger a psoriasis flare-up. Try to maintain normal weight and, if you are dieting avoid crash diets, which can be stressful to the body. Instead take off the weight slowly and sensibly. Bacterial infections, such as strep throat or a yeast infection, may also cause a flare-up. If you have psoriasis, don't let these symptoms go without seeing your physician.

Avoid getting sick—As in many diseases connected to the immune system, if you have psoriasis, don't allow yourself to get rundown. Eat foods rich in vitamin C, vitamin B6, vitamin E, and betacarotene.

Control stress—Since stress can provide the spark that fuels symptoms, stress relief should be a high priority. That's easier said than done, especially since the pain and symptoms of the disease are, in themselves, stress-inducing. But remember that exercise, meditation, biofeedback, yoga, and psychological counseling can all aid in the relief of stress.

Avoid injury—Injury can also aggravate the condition. If you suffer from psoriasis or eczema of the elbows and knees (which are favorite sites for these problems) steer clear of those types of activities such as rollerblading and cycling, on which these areas are at greater risk when there is an accident. Be aware that even resting the elbows on your desk while talking on the phone can irritate those areas.

Oatmeal baths (especially those brands that include a moisturizer) can be helpful in reducing the itching of psoriasis and eczema. If you find oatmeal baths irritating, use a plain bath oil.

Earl's Rx

Vitamin A: Take 10,000 IU with 800 vitamin D daily.

Omega-3 fatty acids: One 1000 mg. capsule three to six times daily.

Selenium: Take 200 mcg. tablet or capsule daily.

Yellow dock: One capsule up to three times daily.

Evening primrose oil: One capsule three times daily.

Sleep Disorders

Sleep disorders represent one of the most common complaints encountered by physicians.

One out of four people in the United States suffers from chronic insomnia.

By age sixty-five, about half of all Americans experience some form of sleep disorder.

For women over forty, sleep disorders are often due to menopausal discomfort.

F ind yourself tossing and turning all night? You're not alone. About 50 million Americans (half of all adults) suffer from sleep problems at one time or another.

Sleep disorders is a broad term that is used to describe everything from insomnia to frequent night wakenings to waking up too early. The two most common types of sleep disorders are *sleep-onset insomnia,* which is characterized by difficulty in falling asleep, and *maintenance insomnia,* which is frequent or early awakening.

Why do so many people have so much trouble doing an activity that is supposed to come naturally? Sleep researchers tell us that approximately 50 percent of all cases of insomnia are due to psychological factors such as depression or anxiety. Clearly, feeling stressed and worried can interfere with our ability to sleep soundly. Some of the other causes of sleep problems may be due to other factors including chronic pain, too much caffeine or alcohol, sleep apnea (breathing problems), muscle spasms and cramps, and various other physical ailments.

If your sleep disorder is related to a physical or emotional problem, common sense dictates that you need to tackle your primary problem before resorting to sleep aids. If stress is making you toss and turn all night, you need to find ways to control it. If you wake up in pain from a muscle cramp, you should seek help from your physician or natural healer. If you load up on caffeine during the day, cutting back on caffeinated beverages may help you have more restful nights. However, if you have a bona fide sleep disorder, there are many things that you can do that will help you get a good night's sleep.

Here is one thing that emphatically I do not recommend: popping a sleeping pill. Millions of people spend billions of dollars on pills and potions that promote sleep. Tranquilizers, antidepressants, and the class of drugs known as *hypnotics* are all used in commercial sleep-aid formulas. Although these drugs may knock you out, many people wake up with "hangovers" that are quite unpleasant. In addition, some of these drugs are addictive, and may even cause some serious side effects such as high blood pressure or impotence. When it comes to sleep, I recommend using only natural remedies.

Natural Hormones

Melatonin—In recent years, there has been a great deal of attention given to *melatonin,* a hormone that is produced by the body, which is reputed to have antiaging properties. Melatonin also helps to regulate sleep cycles and is a veritable cure for insomnia.

Produced in the pineal gland, a peasized structure embedded deep within our brains, it controls the body's circadian rhythm, the internal mechanism that tells us when it's time to sleep and when it's time to wake up.

Melatonin peaks during childhood, drops during adolescence when other hormones kick in, and continues to decrease as we age. By age sixty, our pineal gland is producing half the amount of melatonin it did when we were twenty. One of the most devastating effects of the loss of melatonin is disturbance of sleep patterns.

Researchers have discovered that tiny doses of melatonin supplements are sufficient to bring melatonin blood levels to their normal levels and to induce sleep. It does this by correcting the imbalances in the body's circadian rhythm without resulting in the dependency or side effects typical of sleeping pills.

In one ground-breaking Israeli study at the Technion Medical School in Haifa, researchers gave melatonin supplements at night to men and women between the ages of sixty-eight and eighty. The results were remarkable: Patients on melatonin had less trouble falling asleep (the time required to fall asleep was cut in half!) and stayed asleep longer without waking up. What was even more exciting was the fact that the subjects reported having a more refreshing sleep, and feeling better in the morning. Since the sixty-five-plus population is responsible for consuming nearly one-half of all sleeping pills on the market, melatonin may prove to be a safe and more effective alternative to commercial sleeping aids. (Only take melatonin at night before bedtime.)

If you are a regular aspirin user take note: Aspirin interferes with melatonin secretion, which can interfere with sleep. Therefore, avoid taking aspirin at night. (If you suffer from night terrors, do not use melatonin: Studies have suggested that it may worsen this condition.)

Minerals

Calcium and Magnesium—These two minerals are natural tranquilizers that have a calming effect on the body. Calcium and magnesium have been shown to reduce blood pressure, relieve stress, and ready the body for sleep.

Herbs

Passion flower—Use of this herb dates back to the Aztecs, who first recognized its sedative qualities. Today, passion flower is a popular treatment for sleep disorders and anxiety in Europe. Passion flower is included in many herbal formulas designed to promote relaxation and sleep.

Valerian—For centuries, herbal healers have used valerian as a sedative for the relief of insomnia, anxiety, and conditions associated with pain. Recent scientific studies have substantiated valerian's ability to improve sleep quality and relieve insomnia.

For example, in a double-blind study involving 128 subjects, an extract of valerian root helped participants to sleep better, improved the quality of sleep, and reduced the time required to fall asleep. Even better, it did not leave a telltale "hangover" the next morning.

Kava kava—This herb, a member of the pepper family, has been used for medicinal purposes in the Pacific islands since earliest times. It helps alleviate insomnia through its sedative qualities; a cup of kava tea makes you feel relaxed and pleasantly groggy. Unlike alcohol and other sedatives, kava does not produce any morning hangover.

Chamomile tea—This is my favorite antidote for insomnia! I sip a cup of chamomile tea every night, and never have any difficulty sleeping.

Since it is a member of the daisy family, which also includes ragweed, avoid it if you suffer from hay fever.

Lemon balm—This pleasant-tasting herb has long been used to treat nervous tension and insomnia.

Peppermint—This tea has a soothing effect on the body and may help to promote sleep.

Skullcap—This herb may help to promote sleep by reducing the aches and pains that can keep you up at night. It is often included in herbal sleep formulas.

Personal advice

First, watch the stimulants. Caffeine, which is found in coffee, tea, soft drinks, and chocolate, should be avoided from early afternoon until bedtime. Next, establish a fixed sleep schedule, then stick to it. Don't smoke. Nicotine is a powerful stimulant; that bedtime cigarette may be what's keeping you up at night. If physical ailments are disturbing your sleep, see a physician.

Exercise during the day—walking outdoors is a good way to help control stress, but don't exercise too close to bedtime, since exercise can be a stimulant.

Earl's Rx

If a cup of chamomile or another relaxing herb tea doesn't do the trick, try the following sleepytime formula. I guarantee that you will sleep like a baby!

Calcium and magnesium: These supplements are sold in a combination tablet of calcium (500 mg.) and magnesium (250 mg.) Take up to two tablets one half hour before bedtime.

Melatonin: Take .5–1 mg. before bedtime. I prefer the sublingual form that dissolves under the tongue.

Kava kava: Take one or two capsules at night before bedtime.

If your insomnia is caused by excess stress:

Valerian: Take one capsule up to three times daily.

Passion flower: One or two capsules before bedtime.

Stroke

Stroke is the third leading cause of death in the United States.

Risk factors for stroke include high blood pressure, arteriosclerosis, heart disease, and diabetes mellitus.

The brain is the command center of the body that controls virtually all bodily functions, from breathing to the beating of our hearts to our ability to think and speak. Like other organs of the body, the brain requires a steady flow of blood and oxygen to function normally. When the supply of blood to the brain is impaired, it can cause a *stroke*, a sudden malfunction of the brain. If oxygen levels in the brain drop low enough, there can be permanent neurological damage.

Not all strokes are the same; some are so slight the victim may not even be aware he is having one. In some cases, the person experiencing a stroke may simply feel a slight numbness in his face or arm, or may have difficulty speaking or thinking clearly for a brief period of time. For other people, the stroke is so devastating that it can cause permanent paralysis or even death.

Although all strokes are a result of the reduction in blood flow to the brain, that trigger is not always set off by the same thing. Common causes of stroke include atherosclerosis, blood clots, hemorrhage, and aneurysms.

Atherosclerosis, or the narrowing or blockage of an artery due to fatty deposits, accounts for slightly more than half of all strokes. With proper diet, the right supplements, and a healthy lifestyle, atherosclerosis is a preventable disease. (See "Heart Disease," p. 142.)

In some cases, a stroke will occur if the artery delivering blood to the brain becomes blocked by a blood clot. There are several supplements that can help to prevent blood clots, and I will talk about them later.

In addition, a weakening in the cerebral artery, called an *aneurysm,* could cause an artery to break, thus causing a hemorrhage. Although some aneurysms are genetic, maintaining normal blood pressure can help to prevent arterial weakness that can lead to the formation of an aneurysm. Not smoking also substantially decreases your risk of both aneurysm and stroke.

In many cases, however, strokes can be avoided simply by preventing the underlying medical conditions that leave us vulnerable to them. The following supplements will help to keep you stroke-free.

Vitamins

For several years, doctors have prescribed small doses of aspirin for their patients to help prevent *sticky blood,* or clots that could lead to stroke. New evidence suggests that vitamin E, taken along with aspirin, could enhance aspirin's ability to prevent blood clots. Blood clots are formed by *platelets,* special groups of cells that attach to an artery wall and form clumps. Before the platelet can attach itself to the wall, it must send out a long strand or anchor to hold on to. When enough platelets cling together, a small piece can become unattached from the clump and form a clot. If the clot travels to the artery delivering blood to the brain, it will cause a stroke. One intriguing study suggests that vitamin E and aspirin can thwart the ability of platelets to produce the strands necessary to attach themselves to an artery, thus preventing the formation of clots at the earliest possible stage. In this study, reported in the *American Journal of Clinical Nutrition* (December 1995), one hundred patients who had suffered minor strokes were given either 325 mg. aspirin, or 325 mg. aspirin plus 400 IU of vitamin E, or a placebo, taken daily. After eighteen months, an examination of the patients' blood revealed that the aspirin and vitamin E were much more effective than plain aspirin or the placebo in reducing the number of anchor strands.

(Check with your physician or natural healer before starting aspirin and vitamin E—this therapy may not be advisable for people with very high blood pressure or for those taking blood-thinning medication. Do not exceed recommended doses for E; in megadoses it may actually cause bleeding in some people.)

Carotenoids—Researchers from the Boston-based Nurses' Health Study found that women who ate the most carrots and spinach, foods rich in carotenoids (betacarotene and lutein) had a much lower risk of having a stroke than women who seldom ate these vegetables.

It's not only women, however, who benefit from eating good food. One of the reports to come out of *The Framingham Study,* which followed 832 men age forty-five through sixty-five years for three years suggests that the daily intake of fruits and vegetables may protect against development of stroke in men.

Vitamin A—Evidence that vitamin A may relieve the neurological damage in stroke patients comes from a study in Belgium. Doctors in Brussels measured serum levels of vitamins A and E in eighty people who suffered from middle-cerebral-artery ischemia. The patients who had high blood-concentration levels of vitamin A suffered less neurological damage from their strokes and recovered faster and more fully than the people with low vitamin A levels. The encouraging news is that many people in the first group recovered almost completely within twenty-four hours, and only two had severe disabilities of a result of their stroke.

Doctors speculate that vitamin A works to prevent brain damage because it acts more strongly as an antioxidant in conditions where oxygen levels are low, as they are during a stroke.

Minerals

Calcium and vitamin D—Low calcium and vitamin D intake has been linked to stroke. Researchers compared the diets of thirty-five women who have had strokes accompanied by no history of high blood pressure or heart disease, with the diets of women who have never had strokes. Results indicate that the healthy women's diets contained 38 percent more vitamin D and 17 percent more calcium than those of the stroke victims.

Selenium—This mineral is also synergistic with vitamin E, meaning that the combination of the two is far more potent than either one alone. People who live in areas where the soil is poor in selenium (and therefore is not present in locally grown food and water) have significantly higher incidence of stroke than do people who live in selenium-rich areas. In fact, the southwest United States—known as the *stroke belt* due to its high rate of stroke—is the most selenium-deficient region in the United States. Good food sources of selenium include broccoli, garlic, whole wheat, onions, shellfish, chicken, and red grapes. Selenium is also included in many antioxidant formulas.

Potassium—A study from Temple University in Philadelphia showed that low-potassium diets may be a cause of high blood pressure. Getting plenty of potassium-rich foods like bananas, orange juice, tomatoes, dried apricots, lima beans, and potatoes may be essential for regulating blood pressure.

Herbs

Alfalfa—Animal studies show that alfalfa leaves help reduce blood-cholesterol levels and plaque deposits on artery walls. Additional studies are being conducted to find out if the same effect is true for humans.

Ginger—This plant may help reduce cholesterol, according to a study published in the *New England Journal of Medicine*. It also helps lower blood pressure and prevent the internal blood clots that trigger some strokes.

Gingko biloba—Ginkgo is definitely the herb for your brain and, in addition to improving memory (see "Memory Loss," page 187), it may also protect your brain from the lethal effects of stroke. Recently, scientists discovered that ginkgo can interfere with the action of a substance the body produces called *platelet activation factor* (PAF), which is involved in arterial blood flow. As people grow older, blood flow to the brain can decrease, resulting in less oxygen for brain cells. Dozens of studies show ginkgo significantly increases blood flow to the brain and may even speed recovery from stroke.

Tarragon oil—This oil contains a bioflavonoid (*rutin*) that strengthens capillary walls. Animal studies show rutin helps prevent plaque deposits that can narrow arteries and cause loss of oxygen leading to stroke.

Tumeric—Tumeric has been used in both cooking and healing in India for thousands of years. Its many healing properties are well documented; recent studies show that tumeric may help reduce cholesterol and prevent internal blood clots that trigger stroke.

Other Supplements

Omega-3 fatty acids—Omega-3 fatty acids are found primarily in fish such as salmon, halibut, albacore tuna, bass, sardines, anchovy, and mackerel that feed on omega-3 marine plants. Omega-3s are natural blood thinners that prevent blood clots that can lead to heart attack or stroke.

Sulfides—Sulfides, found in garlic and cruciferous vegetables, help reduce blood pressure and prevent the formation of blood clots, a leading cause of strokes.

Personal Advice

The biggest risk factor for stroke is high blood pressure (see "High Blood Pressure," p. 156). High blood pressure may be lowered through diet, exercise, and weight control, and by limiting alcohol intake.

Smokers are twice as likely as nonsmokers to have a stroke. Stop smoking and you reduce the risk of stroke to the same level as a nonsmoker within five years.

Excess weight strains the circulatory system and increases the risk of diabetes, heart disease, and high blood pressure. Losing weight involves a change in lifestyle, meaning a change in what you eat, how you deal with stress, and how much you exercise.

Get plenty of exercise, lower your intake of salt, fat, and sugar, reduce intake of alcohol and caffeinated coffee, and take steps to lower stress.

Earl's Rx

Try these stroke busters!

Vitamin E: One 400 IU capsule daily, dry form preferred.*

Selenium: One or two (50–100 mcg.) capsules or tablets daily.

Garlic: Two capsules three times daily (aged raw, odorless).

Ginkgo biloba: One or two 60 mg. capsules daily.

Tumeric: Two capsules up to three times daily.

*Check with your doctor or natural healer before taking vitamin E in combination with aspirin or any other blood thinners.

Sunburn

Serious damage from ultraviolet sunlight is a major health risk.

Experts estimate that 80 percent of all skin damage due to aging is caused by overexposure to the sun.

Your skin feels as though it's on fire. Your hands swell, your eyes hurt, you're sick to your stomach, and there is no way to rest comfortably because you can't lie down without hurting. As many of you may already know, I am describing the classic symptoms of a severe sunburn.

If your burn is severe, you should call your physician. Symptoms such as chills, confusion, severe headache, and vomiting are signs that you may have sunstroke in addition to a bad burn and, in some cases, you may require immediate medical attention. If your sunburn is not that severe, however, natural remedies will both relieve the pain and promote healing.

Vitamins

Vitamins C and E—The ultraviolet rays from the sun, *UVA* and *UVB*, are the culprits that cause your skin to burn, and can inflict substantial damage to healthy skin by promoting oxidative damage by free radicals. Recently, researchers tested two antioxidants, vitamins C and E, for their effectiveness in combating UVB and UVA damage and found that the best results were achieved with a combination of the two vitamins. If you have a severe sunburn, I recommend that you increase your intake of both of these vitamins until you are fully healed.

Minerals

Potassium—If you have a bad sunburn, you may also be suffering from dehydration or the loss of fluid and minerals through your sweat. If you are low in potassium, you will feel tired and sluggish. After a day in the hot sun, I recommend that you take extra potassium to help restore this mineral to normal levels. A glass of orange juice or a banana are excellent sources of potassium.

Herbs

Chamomile—Chamomile tea is known for its calming effect and is a natural tranquilizer. Used externally, it is also good for skin inflammations. Brew a cup of chamomile tea; let it cool. Using a sterile piece of surgical cotton, gently dab the cooled tea directly on the burn.

Aloe—A gel made from this herb relieves pain and promotes healing of burns.

Arnica—Arnica lotion promotes healing of wounds. Use daily, on unbroken skin only.

Calendula—A salve and ointment made from this herb is soothing to skin wounds and bruises.

Personal Advice

Prevention is the best medicine—Unless you've been on another planet for the last five years, you know that early exposure to sunburn can mean skin cancer as an adult. Recent studies also confirm that overexposure to direct sunlight can increase the risk of developing cataracts and macular degeneration, two serious eye diseases that can lead to blindness.

Stay away from tanning salons and high sun. If you love the beach, protect yourself! Wear loose clothing, sunglasses, and a sunhat. Slather on that sunblock and, remember, sunburn is entirely preventable. All you have to do is stay out of the sun! When you do go outdoors, wear a sunscreen with a sun protection factor (SPF) of 15 or even higher. Even if you are wearing a waterproof sunscreen, be sure to reapply sunscreen after swimming, or after two hours of exposure. Put on your sunscreen about one-half hour before going out in the sun; it takes a while for the skin to soak it up.

Eat a diet high in antioxidants to help combat the damage to your skin, drink plenty of fluids if you burn easily and, remember, only you can prevent the agony of sunburn!

Caution—Keep in mind that certain medications (Retin A and tetracycline) can increase sensitivity to sunlight. If you are taking any medicine, be sure to ask your physician if it will increase your susceptibility to burns.

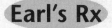

Aloe vera gel can be applied to the skin up to three times daily. If you have a sunburn, these supplements can help promote healing.

Vitamin E: Two 400 IU capsules daily, dry form preferred.

Vitamin C: Three 500 mg. daily of calcium ascorbate with meals.

Potassium: One 99 mg. capsule or tablet up to three times daily.

Taste Loss

Age, medication, and a deficiency in one important mineral can contribute to the loss of taste.

Most of us take it for granted that when we bite into a food that we like we will be able to taste it. Yet for countless numbers of people, food has a bland, off taste, or no flavor at all. In fact, the inability to taste food is a very real problem that can have serious health consequences.

As people age, the loss of taste (and often smell) is a fairly common condition that makes eating a chore as opposed to a pleasure. Studies have shown that older people find it more difficult than younger people to identify sweet, bitter, and salty tastes. No one really knows why this happens, but one theory is that the cells in the nose aren't replaced as efficiently when we are older. Whatever the cause, the inability to perceive flavor is one of the primary reasons that many older people fail to follow a low-fat, fruit and vegetable rich diet that will maintain their energy and health. Very often, people who have lost their sense of taste skip meals or load up on the wrong kinds of food.

When we say a food tastes good, what we really mean is that it smells good, because the two sensations are so closely linked. It is still very much a mystery why some people think certain foods taste good while others cannot stomach the very same items. We do know that when the taste buds are impaired and food has no taste at all, eating becomes a chore. In fact, studies have shown that some obese people lack the ability to fully taste their food and, as a result, they overeat to compensate for that lack, hoping the next bite will be the one with the satisfying taste. Experts also suggest that in some cases, obesity may be due to the fact that foods containing the texture of fat that are also sweet (like ice cream) seem to make up for loss of taste and smell.

We also know that certain poisonous substances and decaying foods have a horrible taste; it may be nature's way of protecting us from eating something that can really harm us.

One man's poison may indeed be another man's meat. For example, people of certain cultures may like foods that other cultures disdain, and this strongly suggests that our tastes can be developed or conditioned starting when we are infants. Remember, when we think we're losing our sense of taste, we may really be losing our sense of smell. That is particularly true when we are suffering from allergies or colds which block the nasal passages, but thankfully these are temporary crises.

Certain medications can also alter the taste of food, or rob it of its flavor. For example, common drugs such as tetracycline, aspirin, steroids, and some tranquilizers affect the taste buds. Fortunately, when these drugs are discontinued, taste sensation usually returns to normal. Obviously, if you are suffering from the loss of taste and are taking any medication on a regular basis, check with your doctor to determine if the drug could be causing the problem.

Diseases ranging from diabetes and Parkinson's to liver disorders and Alzheimer's can also alter both the senses of taste and smell and, as a result, people with these illnesses may be prone to skipping meals, which will leave them in an even more weakened state.

Gender and genetics may also play a part in our ability to taste foods; some people have more taste buds on the tip of the tongue, which means that they may have a sharper sense of taste to begin with and, therefore, can afford to lose a bit without suffering. Women tend to have many more taste buds than men which suggests that sex hormones, including estrogen, play a role in regulating taste perception. A number of studies have shown that taste perception varies with menstruation and pregnancy, and some women lose some taste perception at menopause, or find that foods that they once loved have now become distasteful.

Minerals

Zinc—Zinc deficiency is invariably accompanied by alterations in smell and taste. The same is true for anorexia or for rapid weight loss, which depletes zinc reserves in the body. Recent research indicates that small zinc supplements have shown improvement in taste acuity in some patients suffering from loss of taste.

Personal Advice

Ask your doctor about potential side effects on taste from any prescribed drugs. This might allow you to take the drug after eating, or several hours before eating so it won't interfere with taste or smell.

Wait ten to fifteen minutes after brushing your teeth before eating. Some toothpastes contain chemicals that interfere with taste sensations.

Perk up your food with herbs and spices. Tastes can be developed; try adding extra spices and herbs—the zest may make up for a slight loss of taste, making your meals more appetizing.

Earl's Rx

I recommend a multiple vitamin and mineral supplement with B-complex daily with food for everyone, but it is particularly important for older people who may not be eating as well as they should due to problems such as loss of taste or lack of appetite.

Zinc: Take 15–50 mg. daily.

Teeth and Gum Disease

Half of all adults have gums that bleed.

Better nutrition, better dental hygiene and awareness of the importance of dental care, have all contributed to better tooth health.

Remember those commercials that had youngsters yelling the words "Look Mom, no cavities"? It was one of the most popular advertising campaigns ever, and sold millions and millions of tubes of toothpaste. But toothpaste may be the least important ingredient in insuring good tooth health. A combination of common sense and the right supplements can help to keep your gums healthy and your teeth cavity-free. Dental cavities are caused by the breakdown of sugar in the mouth, which forms an acid that corrodes the tooth enamel. Sugar, candy, and other sweets are the major culprit, but so is any form of carbohydrates, particularly foods that are sticky and lodge inside crevices in the teeth.

Gum problems are also fairly common among adults; in fact, nearly everyone suffers from gum disease at some point in their lives. Gum disease is caused by the same culprit that causes cavities, that is, the accumulation of bacterial plaque. If plaque collects on teeth, it can erode the enamel and cause injury. If plaque occurs near the gum line, it can cause irritation and infection which can cause the gums to recede, or pull away from the teeth. When the gums recede, it leaves pockets of empty space that are quickly filled up by more plaque. In severe cases, the gum and the underlying tissue may become so infected, that one or more teeth may need to be removed.

As we age, we lose bone, and this too can create problems with our teeth. Teeth are attached to the jawbone which, over time, like other bones, can thin out, thus providing less stability for the teeth. It is not uncommon for teeth to loosen as the jawbone shifts, leaving them vulnerable to infection.

In addition as people get older they often develop *dry mouth syndrome,* in which they produce less saliva, and this too, can be detrimental to teeth. Recently, researchers at the Columbia University School of Dentistry found that compounds in saliva actually protect the mouth and teeth from infection by washing out food particles and reducing the ability of bacteria to stick to the teeth, and by fighting bacteria. These compounds also protect the enamel layer of new teeth in children against acids, which can wear it down. If you do not produce enough saliva, however, your run the risk of developing cavities and infections.

Vitamins

Vitamin C and bioflavonoids—Vitamin C and bioflavonoids work together to repair damaged tissue and can help strengthen gums. Rutin is the bioflavonoid renown for its ability to cure bleeding gums.

Folic acid—This B vitamin, which is good for many other things, has also been shown to reduce gum inflammation.

Herbs

Green tea—For centuries, Japanese parents have advised their children to drink green tea after eating sweets. Researchers at the University of California at Berkeley recently learned that flavor compounds called *tannins*, found in green and black tea, can kill the bacteria that are responsible for tooth cavities. Plant tannins also contain highly complex molecules called *catechins*, which bind to gum tissue and tooth surfaces alike, and can prevent plaque accumulation and buildup of plaque organisms on the tooth surface. Green tea is also naturally high in fluoride, a mineral which is essential for strong teeth.

Evening primrose oil—If dry mouth is a problem, this herb can help improve saliva flow.

Minerals

Fluoride—In the 1930s, researchers noticed that there was an inverse relationship between fluoride levels in the drinking water and the prevalence of tooth decay. In the 1950s, many communities across the United States began to fluoridate their drinking water, and the results have been dramatic. In communities where fluoride levels are low, dentists often give patients extra fluoride treatments. If you are living in an area where the water is fluorinated, you are getting enough protection.

If you don't, good food sources of fluoride are seafood, green and black tea, and gelatin.

Calcium and vitamin D—Calcium is the most abundant mineral in the human body, and requires adequate amounts of Vitamin D to be properly absorbed. Roughly 99 percent of the body's calcium is found in teeth and bones. Maintaining good calcium stores in the body is essential to good tooth health. Good food sources include low-fat milk and yogurt, fortified breakfast cereals, salmon and sardines with bones, tofu made with calcium sulfate, blackstrap molasses, and amaranth, a grain that was highly prized by the Aztecs.

Other Supplements

Coenzyme Q10—This supplement helps to strengthen the gums, which are essential for maintaining healthy teeth. CoQ10 bolsters the body's immune system, helping to fight off bacteria that could cause cavities and gum disease.

Personal Advice

Brush carefully—Ever hear the phrase "less is more?" When it comes to brushing our teeth, a lot of us are guilty of just the opposite. That's why we might spend a lot of time using a very hard toothbrush to scrub and scrub in order to better insure clean teeth. That is probably one of the worst things we can do to our mouths. Remember, teeth are made of enamel. If you constantly scrub your enamel pots with a hard brush, you will eventually scrub away the enamel. The same thing can happen with our teeth. Combine a hard toothbrush with a heavy hand and you leave your teeth susceptible to tooth sensitivity and cavities.

It's better to use a soft toothbrush tilted at a 45-degree angle, so that the bristles can reach teeth and gums at the same time. Use small, gentle circular motions as if you were massaging rather than scrubbing your teeth. Brush at least once a day or, even better, twice a day. And don't forget to floss; it is important to get the food that lodges in the mouth out of there before bacteria can latch on to it and do their damage.

Diet tips—As every schoolchild knows, sugar in the mouth encourages cavity-causing bacteria to flourish, therefore, cutting back on sugar really will help reduce cavities. In addition, high-carbohydrate foods that rapidly convert into sugar, such as potato chips and cheese puffs, are major no-nos because they can stick to your teeth. If you eat foods such as dried fruit, which can get into tiny crevices within the teeth, be sure to brush and rinse thoroughly when you are through.

Avoid sucking candies or chewing gum, because the longer the sweet remains in your mouth, the more damage it can cause. Don't sip sugary cola drinks or sweetened beverages; in fact, cut down on total sugar amounts in the diet.

Since calcium is vital to strong bones and teeth and alcohol impairs calcium absorption, limit alcohol intake.

Remember, see your dentist at least once a year: This is one case where an ounce of prevention can mean healthy teeth, and it can also literally mean *keeping* your teeth.

Tip for parents—In babies, a major cause of tooth decay is falling asleep while drinking a bottle full of sweet liquid or milk, because these fluids reduce saliva flow during sleep.

Quick first aid for a tooth ache—Bring on the hot chili peppers! The active ingredient in pepper is capsaicin, which has the ability to block pain sensations. This blocking effect is what makes it a longlasting anesthetic. (Caution: Do not use capsaicin if you have tender or sore gums; it can be irritating.)

Earl's Rx

Vitamin C and bioflavonoids: Take 500–1000 mg. daily with food.

Calcium and vitamin D: Take 1000 mg. of calcium (with 500 mg. of magnesium to maintain the proper mineral balance) and 400 IU of Vitamin D daily.

Coenzyme Q10: One 30–100 mg. capsule daily.

Vaginal Yeast Infections

About 75 percent of women will get a vaginal yeast infection at least once.

For many women, yeast infections are a recurrent problem.

Vaginal yeast infections are one of the most common of all gyneco-logical problems and, although they are not serious, they can be very uncomfortable. Yeast infections are also very persistent and, in many cases, difficult to treat.

Why are yeast infections so common? The vagina is warm and moist, making it the perfect environment for many lively microorganisms. One class of these microorganisms is yeast and, although there are hundreds of different kinds of yeast, the one that causes more than 90 percent of the cases of fungal vaginitis is *Candida albicans.*

There is a delicate balance between pH (acid), glycogen, glucose, carbohydrates, and hormones in the vagina. When that balance is thrown off it gives yeast microbes an opportunity to flourish. Some of the events that can trigger those imbalances include use of antibiotics, oral contraceptives, pregnancy, a weakened immune system, poor nutrition, stress, and illness.

Why do antibiotics breed yeast infections? Antibiotics which are important infection fighters, cannot tell the difference between the good and the bad organisms. Thus, antibiotics encourage yeast growth primarily by killing off the good with the bad, giving existing *Candida albicans* organisms an opportunity to reproduce and colonize.

Women who use oral contraceptives are significantly more likely to suffer from yeast infections than nonusers. The pill causes hormonal changes that alter the acid balance in the vagina, thus allowing the troublesome yeast to multiply. For the same reason, yeast infections are also more common during pregnancy.

Under normal conditions, we have a strong natural immunity to fungal disease agents such as *candida.* Healthy, well-nourished adults with well-functioning immune systems have an innate ability to rid themselves of opportunistic microorganisms like *candida.* Anything that impairs the immune system, like chemotherapy, excessive stress, and illness, gives yeast an opportunity to flourish. Fortunately, there are several supplements that can bolster our resistance against yeast infection.

Friendly Bacteria

Acidophilus—One way to promote a healthy vaginal environment is to introduce good bacterial organisms into the body though the consumption of active acidophilus cultures. Yogurt contains *Lactobacillus acidophilus* (commonly known as *acidophilus*), a friendly bacteria that is used to ferment milk into yogurt and is also present in the gastrointestinal tract.

Recently Dr. Eileen Hilton at the Long Island Jewish Medical Center fed yogurt containing lactobacillus acidophilus cultures for six months to women with a history of chronic yeast infections. Women who ate 8 ounces of yogurt containing live cultures of Lactobacillus acidophilus once a day for six months had three times fewer infections than women who ate no yogurt.

Look for yogurt that bears the National Yogurt Association's "live and active cultures" seal, and avoid yogurt products that are loaded with fruit and sugar. Frozen yogurt contains more fat and sugar, less calcium, and few live-active bacteria. Acidophilus is also sold in capsule form.

Herbs

Echinacea—Research has shown that compounds isolated from echinacea can reduce the rate of growth of *Candida albicans* in the vagina. In a recent German study, 203 women with recurrent vaginal yeast infections were treated with either an antiyeast cream or the cream plus an oral echinacea preparation. After six months, 60 percent of the women treated with just the antifungal cream had experienced recurrences, but among those also treated with echinacea, the figure was only 16 percent. If you have chronic yeast infection, taking echinacea along with your usual treatment may be the way to beat this infection once and for all.

Barberry—This fruit has remarkable infection-fighting properties that kills microorganisms that cause wound infections and vaginal yeast infections.

Chamomile—Long known to soothe jangled nerves, chamomile has also been used for a variety of ailments from fever to indigestion to menstrual discomfort. Studies show the herb kills the yeast fungi *Candida albicans* as well as certain bacteria staphylococcus. Try a cup of chamomile tea at night; it is also a natural sleep aid.

Cinnamon—An infection fighter, it kills disease-causing bacteria and fungi including *candida*. For a good-tasting "antifungal" breakfast, sprinkle some cinnamon on a cup of plain yogurt.

Dandelion—This weed inhibits the growth of the fungus responsible for vaginal yeast infections. Eat some dandelion greens in your salad. Add a couple of handfuls of dried leaves and flowers to your bath water.

Garlic—Researchers at the University of Cambridge in England, found that garlic juice is as strong as the antifungal drugs amphotericin and nystatin, particularly against *Candida*.

Licorice—Many laboratory tests show licorice fights the fungus responsible for vaginal yeast infections. (Do not take licorice orally if you have high blood pressure.)

Other Supplements

Boric acid—Recently, women herbal healers have touted the antiyeast activity of boric acid powder. Rosemary Gladstar, author of *The Woman's Herbal* (a book I believe should be on every woman's bookshelf), offers the following suggestion. Gladstar recommends packing the boric acid loosely into size "o" capsules (available at most health-food stores) and inserting one capsule into the vagina in the morning and again at bedtime for five to seven days. (If you find the treatment to be irritating, discontinue the treatment. The irritation should pass within a day or two.) If you don't want to make up your own capsules, there are pharmacies that will make them up for you.

Tea tree oil—Tea tree oil has been found to be highly effective for the treatment of yeast infections either as a douche or by insertion of a tampon saturated with a solution made from this herb. Tea tree preparations are sold at natural-food stores.

Caprylic acid—Caprylic acid is a saturated fatty acid that has been found to have antifungal activity. It is sold over-the-counter by a number of different companies under various brand names.

Pau D'arco—Also known as *taheebo*, this herb has long been used by the Indians of South America to treat fungal infections of all types.

Personal advice

Starve a yeast infection—Yeast thrive on simple carbohydrates. These include cane and beet sugars, corn and maple syrups and molasses. In the initial stages of yeast infection, avoid foods high in simple carbohydrates and foods with a high content of yeast or mold including alcoholic beverages, cheeses, dried fruits, melons, and peanuts. Limit intake of high carbohydrate vegetables such as potatoes, corn, yams, and parsnips.

Foods that can be eaten freely include all green vegetables and protein sources (legumes, fish, poultry, and meat). Shiitake mushrooms and garlic are good immune boosters. Whole grains, whole wheat, brown rice, peas, beans, and vegetables are more slowly digested and therefore less likely to promote yeast growth.

Yeast infections can be difficult to treat, but simple measures may help to keep them at bay. Wear loose, natural-fiber underwear with cotton crotch. Avoid tights, leggings, pantyhose, and tight jeans. Exercise in breathable clothing. Shower and change right after exercising. Don't sit around in a wet bathing suit, as chlorine in swimming pools can affect the vagina, leading to a chemical-induced irritation that may allow the vaginal yeast to act up. Avoid hot tubs, especially those in public facilities. Wash underwear in very hot water when suffering from yeast infection.

Women should investigate the possibility of having their sexual partners treated with antifungal medications at the same time they undergo treatment, because yeast infections can be passed back and forth between partners. Do not use tampons when an infection is present; they'll absorb antiyeast medication.

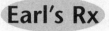

Earl's Rx

Here's some ammunition to help you win the war against yeast infections!

Acidophilus: Take one tablespoon of liquid or one capsule (6 billion organisms) one-half hour before each meal.

Echinacea: One 500 mg. capsule three times daily for two weeks, then one capsule daily for one week.

Garlic: Take 500 mg. of aged raw garlic tablets for three times daily for one month, then one daily thereafter.

Caprylic acid: One capsule three times daily.

Pau D'arco: One capsule three times daily.

Varicose Veins (and Hemorrhoids)

Unsightly and painful, varicose veins are a common problem of aging and inactivity.

Varicose veins are due to a weakness in the wall of the vein, or in the tiny valves that prevent blood from flowing in the wrong direction as it travels up from the legs back to the heart. The veins enlarge and become less efficient, which can allow fluid to leak from the veins back into the tissues of the ankles and feet. Varicose veins can be aggravated by either long periods of standing or sitting, which will cause the blood to pool in one spot. In severe cases, the veins can protrude through the skin and can become quite painful.

Varicose veins can be genetic, but they can also be caused by an excessive strain in the abdominal area (as in the case of pregnancy) and because four times as many women develop varicose veins as men, there is reason to suspect that hormones may play a role.

Hemorrhoids are actually varicose veins in the anus and the rectum, which can cause pain and bleeding. Hemorrhoids are usually caused by excessive straining during bowel movement, most often due to constipation. (For more on preventing constipation, see page 127.)

In severe cases, surgery may be required for varicose veins and hemorrhoids, however, in most cases, supplements can help to keep the symptoms under control.

Herbs

Butcher's broom—This herb is a popular treatment for both varicose veins and hemorrhoids. A salve made from butcher's broom can be used directly on an inflamed hemorrhoid. Taken orally, butcher's broom can help reduce the discomfort caused by varicose veins.

Ginkgo biloba—This herb helps promote good circulation throughout the body, which can help to prevent varicose veins from forming in the first place.

Gotu kola—Natural healers have used this herb for centuries to treat inflammation and swelling due to varicose veins.

Vitamins

Rutin—This bioflavonoid is one of 500 compounds that provide color to citrus fruits and vegetables. Bioflavonoids improve the strength of small blood vessels and capillaries, which can help to strengthen veins, thus preventing varicosities.

Vitamin E—Vitamin E helps to improve circulation to the legs and other extremities.

Personal Advice

Diet tips—If you have hemorrhoids, avoid hot, spicy foods which can be very irritating.

Eat lots of fruits and vegetables that are packed with bioflavonoids that can strengthen blood vessels.

Be sure to get enough exercise daily. A lack of exercise will promote both varicose veins and hemorrhoids.

Earl's Rx

Ginkgo biloba: One 60 mg. tablet or capsule three times daily.

Butcher's broom: One 470 mg. capsule up to three times daily.

Gotu kola: One 500 mg. capsule twice daily.

Rutin: One 500 mg. capsule twice daily.

Vitamin E: Take 400 IU (dry form) three times daily.

Vertigo

Do you remember the sensation you felt after twirling or spinning around when you were a child? When you stopped, remember how the room seemed to swim around you? This is precisely what a vertigo attack feels like. Vertigo is a hallucination. You feel as if you are falling, or spinning around, and the dizzier you feel, the more tightly you root yourself to the ground (either by sitting on the floor or by grabbing the nearest solid object and hanging on for dear life).

Vertigo or dizziness can have several physical causes including dysfunction of the inner ear (the part of the ear that controls balance), brain disorders, eye problems, or even diseases of the gastrointestinal tract or other organs. It can also be caused by hyperventilation brought on by anxiety, or as a result of too much alcohol, a reaction to drugs, or even motion sickness.

If you suffer from dizziness, it's a good idea to see a physician or natural healer who will take the time to thoroughly investigate all possible physical causes. If the physician does not find a specific medical problem, he will usually refer you to an *otologist* (an ear specialist).

The ear doctor will determine if there is disease or tumor of the ear. This is done by subjecting the patient to a variety of tests, none of which are pleasant. That's because the tests are designed to make the patient feel even more dizzy so that a technician can measure eye movements. It's through the measurement of eye movements that determination of the type of vertigo can be made.

If all tests are negative for other medical problems, the diagnosis will most probably be *Meniere's disease* or *Benign Position Vertigo*. (BPV).

Meniere's disease, first identified in 1861 by Posper Meniere, a French physician, is thought to be caused by too much fluid in the inner ear. Attacks of Meniere's disease may occur several times a month or year, and can last from a few minutes to many hours. Some people with this problem experience a spontaneous disappearance of symptoms while others may have attacks for years.

Treatment of Meniere's disease includes several prescription drugs to reduce the feeling of intense motion during vertigo. To control the buildup of fluid, you may also be advised to take a diuretic, a drug that reduces fluid production. A low-salt diet, which reduces water retention, may also be effective.

Benign Positional Vertigo is different from Meniere's disease. As the name implies, it means you feel dizzy when you change position such as getting up from a chair or walking about. Diagnosing the condition is the easy part. The hard part is trying to figure out what's causing the condition and what to do about it. The most common cause is usually a viral infection, which causes an imbalance in the fluid of the ear, although other physical problems such as high or low blood pressure or diabetes may also cause the symptoms.

Treatment of BPV is tricky because there are no drugs specifically designed to correct this imbalance. Motion-sickness drugs are not usually very successful, because these drugs do not cure the condition; at best they only temporarily relieve some of the symptoms. In some cases, patients may be given series of exercises which are designed to reestablish signals from the ear to the brain. These exercises actually are designed to induce feelings of dizziness so that, over time, your brain learns to compensate for whatever is causing the problem. If all else fails, keep in mind that nature heals and, if left alone, vertigo will probably cure itself. However, the symptoms of vertigo are so debilitating that it is often impossible to continue daily life. You can't drive because a dizzy spell while driving may cause an accident, it's difficult to eat because of nausea, walking is difficult, and so forth. Waiting for nature may take months while your job and social life slip away. Here are some other things you can do to speed up the healing process.

Minerals

Calcium and fluoride—Some doctors recommend calcium and fluoride supplements, which are now available in time-release capsules. Why these two minerals should help relieve vertigo is not fully understood. I have heard many anecdotal reports from people who have been helped enormously by this treatment.

Herbs

Ginger—For centuries, healers have been prescribing ginger for dizziness and related problems. A recent study confirmed that ginger's antinausea action has been found to be more effective in relieving motion sickness than the standard motion-sickness drug. According to a report in the British medical journal *Lancet,* motion-sickness was induced in thirty-six volunteers by having them sit in a computerized chair designed to cause seasickness. Some were given ginger powder and some were given the traditional motion-sickness drug. The volunteers were free to stop the chair whenever they felt nausea. Those taking the ginger lasted 57 percent longer than those on the traditional drug.

Ginkgo biloba—For more than five-thousand years, Chinese herbalists have recommended ginkgo for a variety of ailments. Studies show that patients suffering from vertigo experienced dramatic improvement after taking ginkgo, due to increased blood flow to the inner ear.

In one test, researchers studied seventy people with chronic vertigo for three months. Patients were given either ginkgo extract or a placebo. At the end of the study, 18 percent of the people taking the placebo no longer felt dizzy, compared with 47 percent of those who took the ginkgo extract. This study reveals two important things about vertigo. First, as I stated earlier, in many cases it will simply go away regardless of treatment or the lack of it, as it did for some of the placebo takers. It also shows, however, that herbal remedies such as ginkgo can help the body to heal itself.

Vitamins

Vitamin B6—This vitamin is a natural diuretic (which can help to dry up the excess fluid in the ear canal) as well as a antinauseant.

Personal Advice

For thousands of years, the Chinese have been using acupuncture to successfully treat vertigo caused by an imbalance of ear fluid. Acupuncture works by increasing blood flow to the ear. If you are being made miserable by this problem, ask your physician or natural healer about acupuncture.

Earl's Rx

Ginkgo biloba: One 60 mg. three times daily.

Ginger: One 500 mg. capsule two to three times daily.

Vitamin B6: One 50 mg. capsule or tablet up to three times daily with meals.

Wound Healing

Natural remedies, from aloe to ice, are excellent treatments for every-day injuries.

Most everyone has had their share of accidental cuts and burns, from childhood on through adulthood, and most would be considered minor. If you have a serious injury, that is, if you are severely burned or are bleeding profusely, you should call your doctor promptly. In most cases, however, a minor injury will heal quite nicely on its own, and there are numerous natural remedies that can both soothe the pain and promote healing.

For minor burns, nothing works better than cold water or even ice to relieve the hot, stinging sensation typical of these injuries. This home remedy is very effective in both stopping the pain and preventing the injury from worsening, as it often does, as nearby cells become inflamed.

If you have a minor cut, it is best to wash it *gently* with a mild soap, and then to keep the injured area still until the bleeding stops. In some cases, elevating the injured area will also redirect blood flow away from the wound and promote coagulation. If bleeding persists, simply apply pressure to the cut for a few minutes; this will usually stop the bleeding. If the bleeding doesn't stop or is heavy, be sure to call your doctor. (Keep in mind that if you are taking aspirin or any other blood thinner on a regular basis, it will take longer for the blood to clot and for the bleeding to stop.) The following supplements can also help to speed up the healing process.

Herbs

Aloe—Of the more than 600 species of aloe, the most currently popular medicinal variety is aloe vera. Aloe has been renowned for its wound-healing properties as far back as the fourth century B.C, and its benefits are touted in the writings of Hippocrates, the "father" of modern medicine. Legend has it that Cleopatra used aloe gel taken straight from the plant to keep her skin smooth and supple. We rediscovered aloe in 1935, when an American medical journal reported the case of a woman whose x-ray burns were successfully treated with aloe gel. Aloe vera contains a number of compounds necessary for wound healing, including vitamins C and E, two potent antioxidants, and varying amounts of proteins (at least 22 amino acids), complex carbohydrates, glucose, and vitamins and minerals, all of which are essential for the growth of new cells.

Various studies have documented that this herb penetrates injured tissue, relieves pain, is anti-inflammatory and increases the blood supply to the injured area. Aloe may also help to stimulate the growth of new skin.

Some people keep aloe plants at home to provide a readily available source for treatment of burns and other wounds. A wide variety of aloe creams and gels are sold at natural-food stores and I think that one should be in everyone's medicine cabinets.

Calendula—Calendula is an essential oil that can be used externally to soothe burns and promote healing of wounds. Calendula creams are sold in natural-food stores.

Comfrey—This herb was used by the early Greeks and Romans to heal wounds. In the 17th century, English herbalist Nicholas Culpeper recommended comfrey roots for wounds, sores, and broken bones. Comfrey contains *allantoin,* a compound that promotes the growth of new cells. Allantoin is the active ingredient in several over-the-counter skin creams, and prescription skin preparations.

There is some controversy surrounding comfrey because researchers discovered it contains carcinogenic and liver-damaging chemicals, and while it may be advisable to not take this herb internally until further research is available, it is safe and useful when used externally on wounds.

Bromelain—Bromelain is a protein-digesting enzyme group found in pineapple that is also a proven anti-inflammatory that can help to speed up the healing process.

Minerals

Zinc—This mineral, which is essential for the synthesis of protein, helps the body to heal itself and is often recommended for minor cuts and wounds. Skin creams containing zinc are commercially available; zinc is also available in capsules and tablets.

Vitamins

Vitamin E—This vitamin has been used to help heal surgical incisions and can prevent thick scarring. Vitamin E is an anti-inflammatory, and thus will help to prevent the injured area from becoming inflammed. Vitamin E is also an antioxidant and, in this capacity, will help to prevent further oxidative damage to the injury. Vitamin E creams applied directly to a wound can promote healing.

Personal Advice

Don't neglect even the smallest wound or cut. First, wash with soap and water, then apply any of the herbal concoctions discussed. If a wound or sore does not heal within a few days, see your doctor or natural healer, it could be a sign of another problem.

If you anticipate surgery, increase your supply of vitamins C, E, and bromelain to help speed recovery of surgical wounds.

Earl's Rx

If you have a cut or burn, apply aloe, calendula, or comfrey cream as needed. (You can use them together; in fact, there are some special creams that combine all three.) In addition, I recommend taking the following supplements to help Mother Nature do her job.

Bromelain: One 500 mg. tablet three times daily.

Vitamin E: Take 400–800 IU capsule of dry form daily.

Vitamin C: Take 1000–2000 mg. of calcium ascorbate up to three times daily with food.

Zinc: One 15 to 50 mg. tablet daily.

Wrinkles

Wrinkles are the most common sign of aging.

Good skin care begins from the inside out.

Skin is not merely the window dressing that binds us together, it is the largest and hardest-working organ system in the body. Among other things, skin enables the body to retain fluids, helps to regulate body temperature, and provides a protective barrier between potentially harmful substances in the environment and our internal organs. As we age, skin undergoes certain changes, some obvious, some not. First, skin begins to thin and, as a result, becomes less elastic and resilient. In addition, the force of gravity over the years pulls the skin down, making it looser and more flabby.

Underneath the top layers of skin, changes are also occurring that can slowly cause damage. For example, the fine lines and wrinkles which begin to develop during middle age are caused by the breakdown in collagen, the protein that provides support and elasticity of the skin. At the same time, the ability of skin cells to regenerate slows down, resulting in old, tired, dull-looking skin. As we age, the glands of the skin produce less *sebum,* an oily substance that forms a protective coating on the skin, preventing it from becoming dry and flaky.

It is no coincidence that the parts of the skin that are most prone to form telltale lines and wrinkles are those that are most exposed to the sun and outside elements. We used to believe that this was due to the fact that the sun and wind sapped the skin of precious moisture and oil, thus drying it. And at one time, we believed that the solution to wrinkles was simply to apply various face creams that restore moisture. We now know that this approach is far too simplistic. Although the skin does lose moisture through the years, many researchers now feel that the true culprit that causes skin to age are actually free radicals, those overactive oxygen atoms that can wreak havoc among normal, healthy cells.

Free radicals are a normal byproduct of oxygen metabolism. When we are young, our bodies can mount a strong defense against free radicals before they can do much harm, and we produce an abundance of free-radical scavengers and antioxidants which bind to free radicals and neutralize them. As we age, however, our body's defenses weaken, and free radicals are allowed to run amuck. Think of an apple that is cut open and left exposed to the air. Within a short time, the apple becomes oxidized and turns brown. Obviously, it takes free radicals much longer to inflict their damage on our skin, but decades of exposure to open air will exact a steep toll in the form of older, tired-looking skin.

Even if we lived in the healthiest of environments, our bodies would manufacture free radicals on their own. However, few of us live in such pristine surroundings; most of us are exposed to a barrage of chemicals and pollutants that may actually promote the formation of additional free radicals. For example, smog and prolonged exposure to ultraviolet light from the sun, pesticides and other pollutants have been shown to increase free radical production. In addition, tobacco smoke, nicotine, and alcohol can also produce free radicals. Given the fact that we are continually bombarded with free radicals, it is essential that we bolster our defenses against these troublemakers.

Diet, a sensible lifestyle and skin-enhancing supplements can help to keep skin smooth and supple, and wrinkles at bay.

Antioxidants

Vitamin C—Vitamin C is not only a potent antioxidant, but is essential for the formation of *collagen*, the substance that binds together cells of connective tissue. For these reasons, it is a critical vitamin for healthy skin. Vitamin C also boosts levels of glutathione, another antioxidant that protects against free-radical damage.

Vitamin E—Vitamin E is also a powerful antioxidant that can help make skin look better. In one recent study, twenty middle-aged women were given a 5 percent vitamin E cream to put on their skin daily. At the end of four weeks, the women reported a significant reduction in the length and depth of crow's feet (those annoying lines around the eyes,) and generally better-looking skin. There are several vitamin E creams on the market. Do not use the Vitamin E straight from the capsule because it can cause irritation in some people.

Superoxide dismutase (SOD) and wild yam—SOD is an antioxidant enzyme that is often teamed with wild yam, which is an excellent source of betacarotene and other members of the carotenoid family. Betacarotene is converted into vitamin A in the body; vitamin A aids in the growth and repair of body tissues and helps to maintain soft, pliant skin.

Other Supplements

DHEA—DHEA, the hormone that declines with age, can help increase the production of sebum, the natural moisturizer that keeps skin supple.

Nucleic acids—Nucleic acids (DNA and RNA) are present in every cell of the body and are essential for the production of new cells, cell repair, and cell metabolism. As we age, we are less able to produce new cells, and some researchers believe that this decline is due to a drop in the production of nucleic acids or a decline in their efficiency. Researchers theorize that if we take nucleic acid supplements, we may be able to stimulate the formation of new cells. This in turn, would help replace old worn-out skin cells with younger-looking, vibrant new cells.

Personal Advice

Here are some skin savers.

Water, water everywhere—Drink at least eight glasses of filtered water daily to replenish lost moisture.

Steer clear of the sun—Limit exposure to the sun to no more than fifteen minutes daily. When going out, be sure to wear a hat and use a sunscreen of SPF 15 strength. (Many people find the higher strengths to be irritating.)

Diet tips—Eat plenty of fresh fruits and vegetables, they are loaded with antioxidants.

Fight the fat—Maintain normal weight; excess weight will cause skin to sag and wrinkle.

Get enough sleep—There is a reason why it's called beauty sleep. As we sleep, our bodies pump out human growth hormone, which can help to regenerate old, tired cells.

Earl's Rx

Vitamin C: Three 500 mg. capsules or tablets of calcium ascorbate daily.

Vitamin E: Two 400 IU vitamin E dry form tablets or capsules daily.

Betacarotene: One 25,000 IU capsule or tablet daily.

SOD: One tablet or capsule daily.

Wild yam: One 300 mg. tablet or capsule daily.

DHEA: One 25 mg. tablet or capsule daily if you are over forty.

Nucleic acids (DNA and RNA) combination: One 100 mg. tablet of each daily.

Selected Bibliography

Abraham, A.S., Barry A. Brooks and U. Eylath. "The Effects of Chromium Supplementation on Serum Glucose and Lipids in Patients With and Without Non-Insulin Dependent Diabetes." *Metabolism* 41, no. 7 (July, 1992).

al-Hindawi, M.K., S.H. al-Khafaji and M.H. Abdul-Nabi "Anti-granuloma Activity of Iraqi Withania Somnifera." *Journal of Ethnopharmocology* 37, no. 2 (September 1992): 113–116.

Adlercreutz, H., K. Höckerstedt, C. Bannwart, et al. "Effect of Dietary Components, Including Lignans and Phytoestrogens, on Enterophepatic Circulation and Liver Metabolism of Estrogens on Sex Hormone Binding Globulin (SHBG)." *Journal of Steroid Biochemistry* 27, no. 4–5 (1987): 1135–1144.

Adlercreutz, H., Y. Mousavi, and K. Hockerstedt. "Diet and Breast Cancer." *Acta Oncologica* vol. 31, no. 2 (1992): 175–181.

Altura, B., M. Brodsky, R. Elin, et al. "Magnesium: Growing in Clinical Importance." *Patient Care*. (January 15, 1994): 130–150.

American Heart Association. "Aspirin as a Therapeutic Agent in Cardiovascular Disease." (1993).

Anderson, R.A. "Chromium, Glucose Tolerance, and Diabetes." *Biological Trace Element Research* 32 (1992): 19–24.

Axelrod, J. and T. D. Reisine, "Stress Hormones: Their Interaction and Regulation." *Science* 224 (1984): 452–459.

Baggio, E., R. Gandini, A.C. Plancher, et al. "Italian Multicenter Study on the Safety and Efficacy of Coenzyme Q 10 as Adjunctive Therapy in Heart Failure (interim analysis)." *Clinical Investigator* 71:S (1993): 145–149.

Barger-Lux, M.J. and R.P. Heaney. "The Role of Calcium Intake in Preventing Bone Fragility, Hypertension and Certain Cancers." *Journal of Nutrition* 124 (1994): 1406S–1411S.

Barnes, S., C. Grubbs, K.D.R. Setchell, et al. "Soybeans Inhibit Mammary Tumors in Models of Breast Cancer." *Mutagens and Carcinogens in the Diet*. (1990): 239–253.

Belizan, J.M., J. Villar, L. Gonzalez, et al. "Calcium Supplementation to Prevent Hypertensive Disorders of Pregnancy." *The New England Journal of Medicine* 235, no. 20 (November 14, 1991): 1399–1404.

Bellino, F.L., R.A. Daynes, P.J. Hornsby, et al. "Dehydroepiandrosterone (DHEA) and Aging." *Annals of the New York Academy of Sciences* 774 (1995).

Blumenthal, M. "EAPC Files Petitions for OTC Drug Use for Valerian and Ginger." *HerbalGram* 35 (1995).

——— "Echinacea Highlighted as Cold and Flu Remedy." *Herbalgram* 29 (1993): 8–9.

Bone, M.E., D.J. Wilkinson, J.R. Young, J. McNeil, et al. "Ginger Root—A New Antiemetic." *Anaesthesia* 45, no. 8 (1990): 669–671.

Boukaiba, N., C.L. Flament, S. Archer, et al. "A Physiological Amount of Zinc Supplementation: Effects on Nutritional, Lipid and Thymic Status in an Elderly Population." *American Journal of Clinical Nutrition* 57 (1993): 566–572.

Bowman, B.A.B. "Acetyl-Carnitine and Alzheimer's Disease." *Nutrition Reviews* 50, no. 5.

Bradlow, H.L., and J. Michnovicz. "A New Approach to the Prevention of Breast Cancer." *Proceedings of the Royal Society of Edinburgh* 95B (1989): 77–86.

Brown, D. "Topical Tea Tree Oil for Nail Fungus." *Herbalgram* 35, no. 11.

Butterworth, C.E., K.D. Hatch, M. Maculuso, et al. "Folate Deficiency and Cervical Dysplasia." *Journal of the American Medical Association* 267, no. 4 (January 22–29, 1992).

Castleman, M. "Red Pepper Is Hot!" *Medical Selfcare.* (September-October 1989).

Crook, W. G. *The Yeast Connection.* New York: Vintage Books, 1986.

Darlington, L.G., and N.W. Ramsey. "Review of Dietary Therapy for Rheumatoid Arthritis." *British Journal of Rheumatology* 32 (1993): 502–514.

Dorsch, W., M. Ettl, and G. Hein. "Antiasthmatic Effects of Onions. Inhibition of Platelet-Activating Factor-Induced Bronchial Obstruction by Onion Oils." *International Archives of Allergy and Applied Immunology* 82 no. 3–4 (1987): 535–536.

"Drugs for Migraine." The Medical Letter on Drugs and Therapeutics. 37 (March 3, 1995): 943.

"Extract From Kudzu Vine Curbs Alcohol Desire; Diadzein and Diadzein." *The Addiction Letter* Vol. 9, no. 12, (December 1993).

Fackleman, K.A. "Chicken Cartilage Soothes Aching Joints." *Science News* 144 (September 25, 1993): 198.

Feldman, E.B., S. Gold, J. Greene, et al. "Ascorbic Acid Supplements and

Blood Pressure: A Four Week Pilot Study." *Annals of the New York Acad emy of Sciences* 669: (September 30, 1996) 342–344.

Folkers, C., and J. Ellis. "Successful Therapy with Vitamin B6 and Vitamin B2 of the Carpal Tunnel Syndrome and the Need for Determination of the RDAs for Vitamins B6 and B12 for Disease States." *Annals of the New York Academy of Sciences* 585 (1990): 295–301.

Fotsis, T., M. Pepper, H. Aldercruetz, et al. "Genistein, a Dietary Derived Inhibitor of In Vitro Angiogenesis." *Proceedings of the National Academy of Sciences* 90 (April 1993): 2690–2694.

Fulder, S., and J. Blackwood. *Garlic: Nature's Original Remedy.* Rochester VT.: Healing Arts Press, 1991.

Gao, Y.T., J.K. McLaughlin, W.J. Blot, et al. "Reduced Risk of Esophageal Cancer Associated with Green Tea Consumption." *Journal of the National Cancer Institute* 86, no. 11 (June 1, 1994): 855–858.

Garewal, H.S., and S. Schanta. "Emerging Role of B-Carotene and Antioxidant Nutrients in Prevention of Oral Cancer." *Archives of Otolaryngol Head Neck Surgery* 121 (February 1995): 141–144.

Ghannoum, M.A. "Inhibition of Candida Adhesion to Buccal Epithelial Cells by a Aqueous Extract of Allium Sativum (Garlic)." *Journal of Applied Bacteriology* 68, no. 2 (1990): 163–69.

Gillman, M., A. Cupples, D. Gagnon, et al. "Protective Effect of Fruits and Vegetables on Development of Stroke in Men." *Journal of the American Medical Association* 273, no. 14 (April 1995): 1113–1117.

Graf, E. and John W. Eaton. "Antioxidant Functions of Phytic Acid." *Free Radical Biology and Medicine* 8 (1990): 61–69.

Graham, S., R. Hellman, James Marshall, et al. "Nutritional Epidemiology of Postmenopausal Breast Cancer in Western New York." *American Journal of Epidemiology* 134 (1991): 552–566.

Giovannucci, E., E.B. Rimm, G. Colditz, et al. "A Prospective Study of Dietary Fat and Risk of Prostate Cancer." *Journal of the National Cancer Institute* 85, no. 19 (October 1993): 1571–1578.

Glynn, A. S. and D. Albanes. "Folate and Cancer: A Review of the Literature." *Nutrition and Cancer* 22 1994: 101–119.

Hartman, I. "Alpha-Linolenic Acid: A Preventive in Secondary Coronary Events?" *Nutrition Reviews* 53, no. 7 (1995): 194–196.

Harvard Women's Health Watch "Fibromyalgia" (October 1994).

Hashim, S., V.S. Aboobaker, R. Madhubala, et al. "Modulatory Effects of Essential Oils on the Formation of DNA Adduct by Aflatoxin B1 In Vitro." *Nutrition and Cancer* 21, no. 2 (1994): 170–175.

Hatton, D. and D. McCarron. "Dietary Calcium and Blood Pressure in Experimental Models of Hypertension." *Hypertension* 23, no. 4 (1994): 513–530.

Herve, A., R. Pascale, A. Lieury, et al. "Effect of Two Doses of Ginkgo Biloba Extract (EGb 761) on the Dual-Coding Test in Elderly Subjects." *Clinical Therapeutics* 15, no. 3 (1993): 549–558.

Heseker, H., W. Kubler, V. Pudel, et al. "Psychological Disorders as Early Symptoms of a Mild-to-Moderate Vitamin Deficiency." *Annals of the New Academy of Sciences* 669 (September 30, 1992): 352–357.

Hilton, E., H.D. Isenberg, P. Alperstein, et al. "Ingestion of Yogurt Containing Lactobacillus Acidophilus as a Prophylaxis for Candidal Vaginitis." *Annals of Internal Medicine* 115, no. 5 (1992): 353–357.

Hochman, L.G., R.K. Scher, and M.S. Myerson. "Brittle Nails: Response to Daily Biotin Supplementation." *Cutis* 51, no. 4 (1993): 303–305.

Hofferberth, B. "The Efficacy of EGb 761 in Patients with Senile Dementia of the Alzheimer Type, A Double-Blind, Placebo-Controlled Study on Different Levels of Investigation." *Human Psychopharmacology* 9, (1994): 215–222.

Hoffman, R. "Asthma Update." *Newlife* (July/August 1995).

Holloway, W.R., L.J. Grota and G.M. Brown. "Immunohistochemical Assessment of Melatonin Binding in the Pineal Gland." *Journal of Pineal Research* (1985): 235–251.

Hu, G., C. Han, and J. Chen. "Inhibition of Oncogene Expression by Green Tea and (-)Epigallocatechin Gallate in Mice." *Nutrition and Cancer* 24, no. 2 (1995): 205–209.

Hughes, C.L. "Phytochemical Mimicry of Reproductive Hormones and Modulation of Herbivore Fertility by Phytoestrogens." *Environmental Health Perspectives* 78 (1988): 171–175.

Ip, C. and D. Lisk. "Bioactivity of Selenium From Brazil Nut for Cancer Prevention and Selenoenzyme Maintenance." *Nutrition and Cancer* 21, no. 3: 204–212.

Israel, K, Bob G. Sanders, and Kimberly Kline. "RRR a-Tocoheryl Succinate Inhibits the Proliferation of Human Prostatic Tumor Cells With Defective Cell Cycle/Differentiation Pathways." *Nutrition and Cancer* 24, no. 2 (1995): 162–169.

Jacques, P. "Effects of Vitamin C on High-Density Lipoprotein Cholesterol and Blood Pressure." *Journal of the American College of Nutrition* 11, no. 2 (1992): 139–144.

Jain, A., R. Vargas, S. Gotzkowsky, et al. "Can Garlic Reduce Levels of Serum Lipids? A Controlled Clinical Study." *The American Journal of Medicine* 94 (1993): 632–635.

Jariwella, R.J., R. Sabin, S. Lawson, et al. "Effects of Dietary Phytic Acid (Phytate) on the Incidence and Growth Rate of Tumors Promoted in Fischer Rats by a Magnesium Supplement." *Nutrition Research* 8 (1988): 813–827.

Joosten, E., A. van der Berg, R. Reizler, et al. "Metabolic Evidence that Deficiencies of Vitamin B-12 (Cobalamin), Folate, and Vitamin B-6 Occur Commonly in Older People." *American Journal of Clinical Nutrition* 58 (1993): 468–476.

Jyonouchi, H., L. Zhang, et al. "Immunodulating Actions of Carotenoids: Enhancement of In Vivo and In Vitro Antibody Production to T-Dependent Antigens." *Nutrition and Cancer* 21, no. 1 (1994): 48–57.

Jialal, I., C. Fuller, and B. Huet. "The Effect of a-Tocopherol Supplementation on LDL Oxidation: A Dose Response Study." *Arteriosclerosis, Thrombosis and Vascular Biology* 15, no. 2 (1995): 190 198.

Julius, M., C.A. Lang, L. Gleiberman, et al. "Glutathione and Morbidity in a Community-Based Sample of Elderly." *Journal of Clinical Epidemiology* 47, no. 9 (1994): 1021–1026.

Kamikawa, T., A. Kobayashi, T. Yamashita, et al. "Effects of Coenzyme Q 10 on Exercise Tolerance in Chronic Stable Angina Pectoris." *American Journal of Cardiology* 56 (1985): 247 251.

Kennedy, A.R., P.C. Billings, P.A. Maki, et al. "Effects of Various Preparations of Dietary Protease Inhibitors on Oral Carcinogenesis in Hamsters induced by DMBA." *Nutrition and Cancer* 19 (1993): 191–200.

"Kidney Stones: Rating What You Drink." *Science News.* 149, no. 9 (March 2, 1996): 143.

Krueger, G.C., P.R. Bergstresser, N.J. Lowe, et al. "Psoriasis." *Journal of the American Academy of Dermatology* 11, no. 5, part 2 (1984): 937–947.

Kulkarnia, R.R., P.S. Patki, V.P. Jog, et al. "Treatment of Osteoarthritis with a Herbomineral Formulation: a Doubleblind, Placebo-Controlled, Cross-Over Study." *Journal of Ethnopharmacology* 33 no. 1–2 (May–June 1991): 91–95.

Kunc, G.A., S. Bannerman, B. Field, et al. "Diet, Alcohol, Smoking and Serum B-Carotene and Vitamin in Male Nonmelanocytic Skin Cancer Patients and Controls. *Nutrition and Cancer* 18 (1992): 237–244.

Leaf, A. "Health Claims: Omega-3 Fatty Acids and Cardiovascular Disease." *Nutrition Reviews* 50, no. 5: 150–153.

Lipkin, R. "Vegemania: Scientists Tout the Health Benefits of Saponins." *Science News* 148 (December 9, 1995): 392–393.

Lipkin, R. "Herbal Agent Limits Alcohol Absorption." *Science News* 148 (August 26, 1995): 135.

Lissoni, P., S. Barni, G. Tancini, et al., "A Study of the Mechanisms Involved in the Immunostimulatory Action of the Pineal Hormone in Cancer Patients." *Oncology* 50 (1993): 399–402.

Longcope, C. "Relationships of Estrogen to Breast Cancer, of Diet to Breast Cancer and of Diet to Estradiol Metabolism." *Journal of the National Cancer Institute* 82, no. 11 (June 6, 1990).

Maestroni, G. J. M., A. Conti, and W. Pierpaoli, "Melatonin, Stress, and the Immune System," *Pineal Research Reviews* 7 (1989): 203–226.

Mata, P., L. Alvarez-Sala, M. Rubio, et al. "Effects of Long-Term Monoun-saturated-vs. Polyunsaturated-Enriched Diets on Lipoproteins in Healthy Men and Women." *American Journal of Clinical Nutrition* 55, (1992): 546–50.

Mathew, B., R. Sankaranarayanan, P. Padmanabhan, et al. "Evaluation of Chemoprevention of Oral Cancer With Spirulina Fusiformis." *Nutrition and Cancer* 24, no 2 (1995): 198–202.

Matsukawa, Y.N., N. Marui, T. Sakai, et al. "Genistein Arrests Cell Cycle Progression at G2-M." *Cancer Research* 53 (1993): 1328–1331.

Mayne, S.T., D.T. Janerich, P. Greenwald, et al. "Dietary Beta Carotene and Lung Cancer Risk in Nonsmokers." *Journal of the National Cancer Institute* 86, no. 1 (January 5, 1994): 33–38.

Messina, M., V. Persky, D.R. Setchell, and S. Barnes. "Soy Intake and Cancer Risk: A Review of the In Vitro and In Vivo Data." *Nutrition and Cancer* 21, no. 2 (1994).

Meydani, M. "Vitamin E." *The Lancet* 435 (January 21, 1995): 170–175.

Meydani, M., J.M. Evans, G. Handelman, et al. "Antioxidant Response to Exercise-Induced Oxidative Stress by Vitamin E." *Annals of New York Academy of Sciences* 669 (September 30, 1992): 363–364.

Mindell, E. *Sexual Fitness.* Potomac, Md.: Phillips Publishing, 1993.

Morales, A.J., J.J. Nolan, J.C. Nelson, et al. "Effect of Replacement Dose of DHEA in Men and Women of Advancing Age." *Journal of Clinical Endorcrinology Metabolism* 78 (1994): 1360–1367.

Mowrey, D.B. *The Scientific Validation of Herbal Medicine.* New Canaan, Conn.: Keats Publishing, 1994.

Newsome, D. "Oral Zinc in Macular Degeneration." *Archives of Ophthalmology* 106, no. 2 (February, 1988): 192–198.

Nielson, F. "Studies on the Relationship Between Boron and Magnesium Which Possibly Affects the Formation and Maintenance of Bones." *Magnesium Trace Elements* 6 (1991): 61–69.

Oyama, Y., P.A. Fuchs, N. Katayama, et al. "Myricetin and Quercetin, the Flavonoid Constituents of Ginkgo Biloba, Greatly Reduce Oxidative Metabolism in Both Resting and Ca2-Loaded Brain Neurons." *Brain Research* 635 (1994): 125–129.

Penn, N.D., L. Purkin, J. Kelleher, et al. "The Effect of Dietary Supplementation with Vitamins A,C, and E on Cell-Mediated Immune Function in Elderly Long-Stay Patients: A Randomized Controlled Trial." *Age and Ageing* 20 (1991): 169–174.

Peterson, G. and S. Barnes. "Genistein Inhibition of the Growth of

Human Breast Cancer Cells: Independence From Estrogen Receptors and the Multi-Drug Resistance Gene." *Biochemical and Biophysical Research Communications* 179, no. 1 (August 30, 1991).

Phelps, S. and W. Harris. "Garlic Supplementation and Lipoprotein Oxidation Susceptibility." *LIPIDS* 28, no. 5 (1993): 475–477.

Piyathilake, C.J., M. Macaluso and Jean R. Hine. "Local and Systematic Effects of Cigarette Smoking on Folate and Vitamin B-12." *American Journal of Clinical Nutrition* 60 (1994): 559–66. 1994.

Press, R., J. Geller, and G. Evans. "The Effect of Chromium Picolinate on Serum Cholesterol and Apolipoprotein Fractions in Human Subjects." *The Western Journal of Medicine* 152 no. 1 (January 1990).

Pryor, W.A. "Can Vitamin E Protect Humans Against the Pathological Effects of Ozone in Smog?" *American Journal of Clinical Nutrition* 53 (1991): 702–722.

Ravitzky, M. "Psoriasis." *Newlife* (1995).

Regelson, W. and M. Kalimi. "Dehydroepiandrosterone (DHEA) A Pleiotropic Steroid. How Can One Steroid Do So Much?" In *Advances in Anti-Aging Medicine*, 1, Ronald M. Klatz, ed. 287–317. Larchmont, N.Y.: Mary Ann Liebert, Inc., 1996.

Reiter, R.J. "Pineal Melatonin: Cell Biology of Its Synthesis and of Its Physiological Interactions." *Endocrine Reviews* 12 (1991): 151–180.

Reiter, R.J., D.X. Tan, B. Poeggerler, et al. "Melatonin as a Free Radical Scavenger: Implications for Aging and Age-Related Diseases." *Annals of the N.Y. Academy of Sciences* 719 (1994): 1–12.

Rimm, E., M. Stampfer, A. Ascherio, et al. "Vitamin E. Consumption and the Risk of Coronary Heart Disease in Men." *The New England Journal of Medicine.* Vol 328 (20) 1450–1456. 1993.

Rall, L. and S. Meydani. "Vitamin B 6 and Immune Competence." *Nutrition Reviews* 51, no. 8 (1993): 217–225.

Roebothan, B.V. and R.K. Chandra. "Relationship Between Nutritional Status and Immune Function of Elderly People." *Age and Ageing* 23 (1994): 49–53.

Rose, D. "Dietary Fiber, Phytoestrogens and Breast Cancer." *Nutrition* 8, no. 1 (January/February 1992): 47–51.

Rose, D.P., M. Goldman, and J. Connolly. "High-fiber Diet Reduces Serum Estrogen Concentrations in Premenopausal Women." *American Journal of Clinical Nutrition* 54 (1991): 520–525.

Rosenberg, I. and J.W. Miller. "Nutritional Factors in Physical and Cognitive Functions of Elderly People." *American Journal of Clinical Nutrition* 55 (1992): 1237S–1243S.

Schmidt, K. "Antioxidant Vitamins and B-Carotene: Effects on Immunocompetence." *American Journal of Clinical Nutrition* 53 (1991): 383S–385S.

Seddon, J., U. Ajani, and R.D. Sperduto, et al. "Dietary Carotenoids, Vitamins A,C, and E, and Advanced Age-Related Macular Degeneration." *Journal of the American Medical Association* 272, no. 18 (1994): 1413–1420.

Seelig, M. "Interrelationship of Magnesium and Estrogen in Cardiovascular and Bone Disorders, Eclampsia, Migraine and Premenstrual Syndrome." *Journal of the American College of Clinical Nutrition* 12, no. 4 (1993): 442–458.

Selhub, J., P. Jacques, and P. Wilson. "Vitamin Status and Intake as Primary Determinants of Homocysteinemia in an Elderly Population." *Journal of the American Medical Association* 270 (December 8, 1993): 22.

Shibata, A., T.M. Mack, A. Paganini-Hill, et al. "A Prospective Study of Pancreatic Cancer in the Elderly." *Internal Journal of Cancer* 58 (1994): 46–49.

Shirama, K., T. Furuya, Y. Takeo, et al., "Direct Effect of Melatonin on the Accessory Sexual Organs in Pinealectomized Male Rats Kept in Constant Darkness." *Journal of Endocrinology* 95 (1982): 87–94.

Siani, A., P. Strazzullo, and A. Giacco. "Increasing the Dietary Potassium Intake Reduces the Need for Antihypertensive Medication." *Annals of Internal Medicine*. Vol. 115: 753–759. 1991.

Simopoulos, A. "Omega-3 Fatty Acids in Health and Disease and in Growth and Development." *American Journal of Clinical Nutrition* 54 (1991): 438–463.

Smigel, K. "Vitamin E Moves On Stage in Cancer Prevention Studies." *Journal of the National Cancer Institute* 84, no. 13 (July 1, 1992): 996–997.

Souetre, E., N. Rosenthal, and J.P. Ortonne. "Affective disorders, light and melatonin." *Photodermatology* 5 (1988): 107–109.

"Special Diet Can Help Relieve Symptoms of Gout." *Environmental Nutrition* (September 1992).

Sperduto, R.H., Milton Tian-Sheng, and C. Roy. "The Linxian Cataract Study: Two Nutrition Intervention Trials." *Archives of Opthalmology* 111 (September 1993): 1246–1253.

"St. John's Wort Treats Depression." *Research Reviews: Herbalgram* 33 (1995): 15.

Stampfer, M., C. Hennekens, J. Manson, et al. "Vitamin E. Consumption and the Risk of Coronary Disease in Women." *The New England Journal of Medicine* 328, no. 20 (1993): 1444–1449.

Stephens, N.G., A. Parsons, P.M. Schofield, et al. "Randomized Controlled

Trial of Vitamin E in Patients with Coronary Disease: Cambridge Heart Antioxidant Study (CHAOS)." *The Lancet* 347, no. 9004 (March 23, 1996): 781–786.

Street, D., G. Comstock, R. Salkeld, et al. "Serum Antioxidants and Myocardial Infarction." *Circulation* 90, no. 3 (1994): 1154–1161.

Sugie, Sh., K. Okamoto, T. Tanaka, et al. "Effect of Fish Oil on the Development of AOM-Induced Glutathione S-Transferase Placental Form Positive Hepatocellular Foci in Male F344 Rats." *Nutrition and Cancer* 24, no. 2 (1995): 188–195.

Troiani, M.E., R.J. Reiter, M.K. Vaughan, et al. "Swimming Depresses Nighttime Melatonin Content without Changing N-Acetyltransferase Activity in the Rat Pineal Gland." *Neuroendocrinology* 47 (1988): 55–60.

Tucker, D., James G. Penland, H. Sandstead, et al. "Nutrition Status and Brain Function in Aging." *American Journal of Clinical Nutrition* 52 (1990): 93–102.

Tufts University. "Gray Matter." *Tufts University Diet & Nutrition Letter* 13, no. 7 (September 1995).

Tufts University. "On Cranberry Juice and Urinary Tract Infections." *Tufts University Diet and Nutrition Letter* 12, no. 3. (May 1994).

Tufts University. "Will Eating Less Fat Lower Breast Cancer Risk After All?" *Tufts University Diet and Nutrition Letter* 14, no. 2 (April 1996).

United States Department of Agriculture. *Food and Nutrition Research Briefs* (April–June 1993).

United States Department of Agriculture. *Food and Nutrition Research Briefs* (Jan.–March 1993).

United States Department of Agriculture. *Food and Nutrition Research Briefs* (July–October 1992).

United States Department of Health and Human Services. "Headache: Hope Through Research" NIH Publication no. 84–158 (September 1984).

van den Brandt, P.A., A. R. Goldbohm, P. van't Veer, et al. "A Prospective Cohort Study on Selenium Status and the Risk of Lung Cancer." *Cancer Research* 53 (October 15, 1993): 4860–4868.

van Papendorp, D.H., H. Coetzer, and M.C. Kruger. "Biochemical Profile of Osteoporotic Patients on Essential Fatty Acid Supplementation." *Nutrition Research* 15, no 3 (1995): 325–334.

Varma, S. "Scientific Basis for Medical Therapy of Cataracts by Antioxidants." *American Journal of Clinical Nutrition* 53 (1991): 335S–345S.

"Vitamin B6 and Immune Function in the Elderly and HIV-seropositive Subjects." *Nutrition Reviews* 50, no. 5. (1992): 145–147.

Waldhauser, F., B. Ehrhart and E. Forster. "Clinical Aspects of the Melatonin

Action: Impact of Development, Aging, and Puberty, Involvement of Melatonin in Psychiatric Disease and Importance of Neuroimmunoendocrine Interactions." *Neuroimmunology Review* (1993): 671–681.

Walsh, N., S. Ramamurthy, L. Schoenfeld, et al. "Analgesic Effectiveness of D-Phenylalanine in Chronic Pain Patients." *Archives of Physical Medicine Rehabilitation* 67 (1986): 436–439.

"Why Do Hamsters Stay on the Wagon?" *Science News* 148. 200. September 23, 1995.

Whitteman, J., D. Grobbee, and F. Derkx. "Reduction of Blood Pressure With Oral Magnesium Supplementation in Women With Mild to Moderate Hypertension." *American Journal of Clinical Nutrition* 60 (1994): 129–135.

Wutian, W., Y. Chen, and R.J. Reiter. "Day-Night Differences in the Response of the Pineal Gland to Swimming Stress." *Proceedings of the Society for Experimental Biology and Medicine* 187 (1988): 315–319.

Yang. C.S., and Z. Wang. "Tea and Cancer." *Journal of the National Cancer Institute* 85, no. 13 (July 7, 1993): 1038–1049.

Yoakum, R. "Nightwalkers: Do Your Legs Seem to Have a Life of Their Own?" *Modern Maturity* (September–October 1994).

Zhu Xiao-Dong and Xi-Can Tang. "Improvement of Memory in Mice by Huperzine A and Huperzine B." *Acta Pharmacological Sinica* 6 (November 8, 1988): 492–497.

Ziegler, R. "Vegetables, Fruits and Carotenoids and the Risk of Cancer." *American Journal of Clinical Nutrition* 53 (1991): 251S–259S.

Zupke, M.P. "Should You Worry About Anemia? What to Do if You're at Risk?" *Environmental Nutrition* 16, no. 12 (December 1993).

Index

57 grams of soy protein / day